# Japan and Global Health

Daisuke Akimoto

# Japan and Global Health

Human Security Agenda in the COVID-19
Pandemic

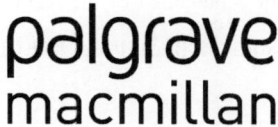

Daisuke Akimoto
Tokyo, Japan

ISBN 978-981-97-0971-7      ISBN 978-981-97-0972-4   (eBook)
https://doi.org/10.1007/978-981-97-0972-4

Cover illustration: © Melisa Hasan

This Palgrave Macmillan imprint is published by the registered company Springer Nature
Singapore Pte Ltd.
The registered company address is: 152 Beach Road, #21-01/04 Gateway East, Singapore
189721, Singapore

Paper in this product is recyclable.

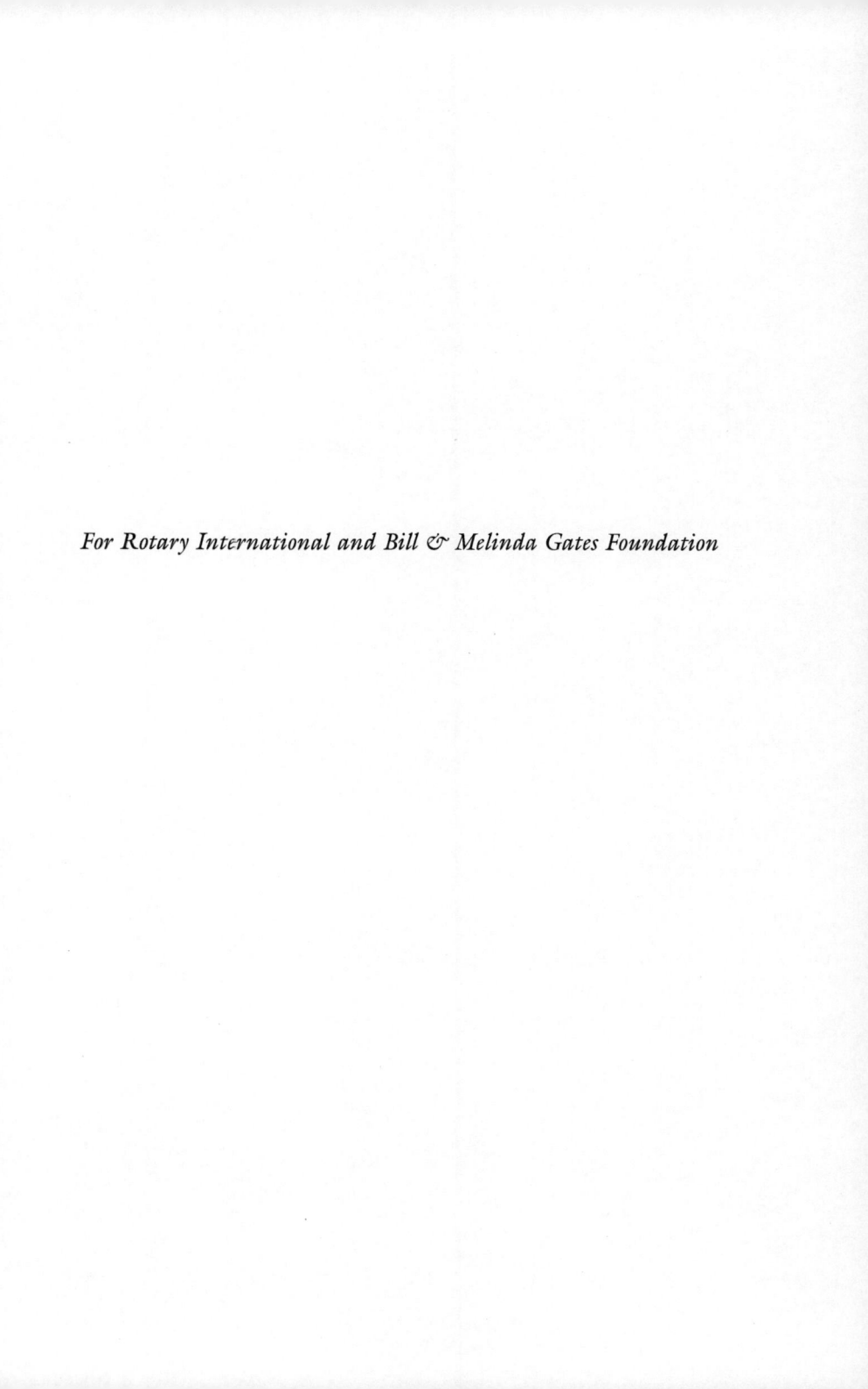

*For Rotary International and Bill & Melinda Gates Foundation*

# CONTENTS

# ABBREVIATIONS

| | |
|---|---|
| ACT-A | Access to COVID-19 Tools Accelerator |
| AI | Artificial Intelligence |
| AIDS | Acquired Immunodeficiency Syndrome |
| AMC | Advance Market Commitment |
| AMR | Antimicrobial Resistance |
| CDC | Centers for Disease Control and Prevention |
| CEPI | Coalition for Epidemic Preparedness Innovations |
| COVAX | COVID-19 Vaccines Global Access |
| DAC | Development Assistance Committee |
| DNDi | Drugs for Neglected Diseases initiative |
| DPJ | Democratic Party of Japan |
| FOIP | Free and Open Indo-Pacific |
| G7/G8 | Group of Seven/Group of Eight |
| GATT | General Agreement on Tariffs and Trade |
| Gavi | Global Alliance for Vaccines and Immunization |
| GFF | Global Financing Facility for Women, Children and Adolescents |
| GHA | Global Health Architecture |
| GHEC | Global Health Emergency Corps |
| GHIT | Global Health Innovative Technology |
| GPEI | Global Polio Eradication Initiative |
| HDI | Human Development Index |
| HGPI | Health and Global Policy Institute |
| HIV | Human Immunodeficiency Virus |
| IBRD | International Bank for Reconstruction and Development |
| ICT | Information and Communication Technology |

| | |
|---|---|
| IDA | International Development Association |
| IFFIm | International Finance Facility for Immunization (Company) |
| IMF | International Monetary Fund |
| IPV | Inactivated Poliovirus Vaccine |
| IWAI | Impact-Weighted Accounts Initiative |
| JAGNTD | Japan Alliance on Global Neglected Tropical Disease |
| JAHSS | Japan Association for Human Security Studies |
| JCIE | Japan Center for International Exchange |
| JICA | Japan International Cooperation Agency |
| LDP | Liberal Democratic Party |
| MCMs | Medical Countermeasures |
| MDGs | Millennium Development Goals |
| MNMJ | Malaria No More Japan |
| NCDs | Non-Commutable Diseases |
| NTDs | Neglected Tropical Diseases |
| ODA | Official Development Assistance |
| OECD | Organization for Economic Cooperation and Development |
| OPV | Oral Poliovirus Vaccine |
| PCR | Polymerase Chain Reaction |
| PHEIC | Public Health Emergency of International Concern |
| PPR | Prevention, Preparedness, and Response |
| R&D | Research and Development |
| RMNCAH-N | Reproductive, Maternal, Newborn Child, Adolescent Health, and Nutrition |
| SCARDA | Strategic Center of Biomedical Advanced Vaccine Research and Development for Preparedness and Response |
| SDGs | Sustainable Development Goals |
| TICAD | Tokyo International Conference on African Development |
| UHC | Universal Health Coverage |
| UNCLOS | United Nations Convention on the Law of the Sea |
| UNDP | United Nations Development Program |
| UNICEF | United Nations Children's Fund |
| VAPP | Vaccine-Associated Paralytic Poliomyelitis |
| WHO | World Health Organization |

# LIST OF FIGURES

# LIST OF TABLES

# CHAPTER 1

# Introduction: Japan and Global Health in the COVID-19 Pandemic

**Abstract** Japan's global health policy was stimulated by the outbreak of a coronavirus pandemic. In the field of global health and human security studies, researchers and experts have published quite a few articles and books in the COVID-19 pandemic. Still, a research gap in the field of Japan's global health policy lies in the fact that there are few book publications on Japan and global health in English despite the significance of this research case in the coronavirus pandemic era. Accordingly, this book attempts to fill in this research gap and examine the development of Japan's global health policy. This chapter intends to contextualize Japan's global health policy in terms of its human security diplomacy, trace Japan's response to the coronavirus pandemic, and clarify the development of Japan's global health strategy during the initial stage of the pandemic period. Finally, it will briefly outline contents of the following chapters.

**Keywords** Coronavirus (COVID-19) · Global health · Human security · Japan · Pandemic

© The Author(s), under exclusive license to Springer Nature Singapore Pte Ltd. 2024
D. Akimoto, *Japan and Global Health*,
https://doi.org/10.1007/978-981-97-0972-4_1

## INTRODUCTION

Japan's global health policy was stimulated by the outbreak of a coronavirus pandemic. In the field of global health and human security studies, researchers and experts have published quite a few articles and books in the COVID-19 pandemic. For instance, Rajib Shaw and Anjula Gurtoo co-edited a book on human security agenda during the global pandemic in terms of development and technology, including response to climate change, poverty, urban–rural linkages, international migration, food systems, water usage, education, gender issue, green infrastructure, transportation system, etc.[1] Anders Granmo and Pieter Fourie focused on health norms and global governance of development, paying attention to COVID-19, Ebola, and HIV/AIDS (human immunodeficiency virus/acquired immunodeficiency syndrome), in the coronavirus pandemic period.[2]

Eddy Elahi shed light on the role of nonprofit organizations as actors of global health,[3] and non-governmental organizations, such as the Bill & Melinda Gates Foundation (Gates Foundation), which have exerted profound influence over the global health policies around the globe. As a matter of fact, billionaire philanthropist Bill Gates authored a book, *How to Prevent the Next Pandemic*, in which he suggested to control early stage of pandemic so that the next possible pandemic could be prevented in the post-COVID-19 pandemic era.[4] Bill Gates has warned that "The world did not prioritize global health until it was too late, and the result has been catastrophic. Countries failed to prepare for pandemics, rich countries reduced funding for R&D, and most governments failed to strengthen their health systems. Although we're finally reaching the light at the end of the tunnel, COVID still kills several thousand people every day".[5]

[1] Shaw, Rajib and Anjula Gurtoo, eds. 2022. *Global Pandemic and Human Security: Technology and Development Perspective*. Singapore: Springer.

[2] Granmo, Anders and Pieter Fourie. 2021. *Health Norms and the Governance of Global Development: The Invention of Global Health*. New York: Routledge.

[3] Elahi, Ebby. 2020. *Insights in Global Health: A Compendium of Healthcare Facilities and Nonprofit Organizations*. Oxon: Taylor & Francis Group.

[4] Gates, Bill. 2022. *How to Prevent the Next Pandemic*. New York: Knopf.

[5] Gates, Bill. May 2022. "No More Pandemics". https://www.gatesnotes.com/How-to-Prevent-the-Next-Pandemic.

In Japan, the Japan Center for International Exchange (JCIE) published a research paper, "Japan's Global Health Diplomacy in the Post-COVID Era".[6] The JCIE paper made a proposal that "Japan should aim to double the funding directed to global health activities from both the public and private sectors in the next five years".[7] Leading Japanese scholars of global health policy, such as Hideaki Shiroyama, Ayako Takemi, Yasushi Katsuma, Makiko Matsuo, Satoshi Ezoe, Kayo Takuma, and Kenichi Doi, published a book on "global health governance" in the middle of the COVID-19 pandemic.[8] Specifically, Satoshi Ezoe as Director of Global Health Policy Division, International Cooperation Bureau, in the Ministry of Foreign Affairs emphasized the significance of global health and universal health coverage (UHC) by referring to Access to COVID-19 Tools Accelerator (ACT-A). The ACT-A as an international framework was established by nine countries and regions including Japan, the World Health Organization (WHO), and the Gates Foundation in April 2020.[9]

A research gap in the field of Japan's global health policy lies in the fact that there are few book publications on Japan and global health in English despite the significance of this research case in the coronavirus pandemic era. Accordingly, this book attempts to fill in this research gap and examine the development of Japan's global health policy, especially paying attention to Japan's response to the COVID-19 pandemic. To this end, this research investigates Japanese politics in the light of global health, and this approach can be categorized as a study of "global health politics".[10] In the light of the study of global health politics, this chapter intends to contextualize Japan's global health policy in terms of its human security diplomacy, trace Japan's response to the coronavirus pandemic,

[6] Japan Center for International Exchange (JCIE). 2020. "Japan's Global Health Diplomacy in the Post-COVID Era: The Paradigm Shift Needed on ODA and Related Policies: Recommendations". https://www.jcie.org/wp-content/uploads/2020/12/Overview-report-e-122120.pdf.

[7] Ibid., p. 6.

[8] Shiroyama, Hideaki, ed. 2020. *Global Health Governance*. Tokyo: Toshindo Publishing.

[9] Ezoe, Satoshi. 2021. "Toward New Solidarity in Global Health: Universal Health Coverage and Reform at the WHO". *Discuss Japan: Japan Foreign Policy Forum*. No. 67, pp. 1–7. https://www.japanpolicyforum.jp/pdf/2021/no67/DJweb_67_dip_02.pdf.

[10] McInnes, Colin, Kelley Lee, and Jeremy Youde, eds. 2020. *The Oxford Handbook of Global Health Politics*. Oxford: Oxford University Press.

and clarify the development of Japan's global health strategy during the initial stage of the pandemic period. Finally, it will briefly outline contents of the following chapters.

## THE DEVELOPMENT OF JAPAN'S HUMAN SECURITY DIPLOMACY

In response to the outbreak of COVID-19, the Shinzo Abe government was forced to tackle the spread of the virus by quarantining the Diamond Princess cruise ship (which at the beginning of its quarantine had ten infected people on board), calling for school closures, conducting travel restrictions from overseas countries, as well as encouraging citizens to stay home and telework.[11] Meanwhile, from April 3, 2020, the US embassy in Tokyo urged American citizens in Japan to return to the United States as soon as possible. It was explained that a test of "polymerase chain reaction" (PCR) to test potentially infected people for the virus was unavailable and insufficient in Japan, and that it was difficult to accurately account for the real number of positive cases in Japan.[12]

On April 7, 2020, Prime Minister Abe announced a national state of emergency in seven cities including Tokyo, yet the measures were criticized as slow and indecisive both domestically and internationally.[13] Given the casualties around the rest of the world, it is no exaggeration to say that the spread of COVID-19 is a crisis in "human security".[14] In the middle of the unprecedented human security crisis that the coronavirus pandemic has wrought, it has been critical for the Japanese government to both save lives and simultaneously facilitate international cooperation in the global

[11] Szechenyi, Nicholas and Joseph S. Bermudez Jr. April 23, 2020. "Japan's Response to Covid-19: A Work in Progress". *CSIS Commentary*. https://www.csis.org/analysis/japans-response-covid-19-work-progress.

[12] Akiyama, Shinichi. April 4, 2020. "US Embassy in Japan Urges Citizens to Return Home, Citing Lack of Virus Testing". *Mainichi Shimbun*. https://mainichi.jp/english/articles/20200404/p2a/00m/0in/014000c.

[13] Walton, David and Daisuke Akimoto. April 7, 2020. "Japan and Coronavirus: Abe Needs to Make Bold Decisions". *The Interpreter*. https://www.lowyinstitute.org/the-interpreter/japan-and-coronavirus-abe-needs-make-bold-decisions.

[14] Fukushima, Akiko. April 16, 2020. "COVID-19 Is a Human Security Crisis". *East Asia Forum*. https://www.eastasiaforum.org/2020/04/16/covid-19-is-a-human-security-crisis/.

health sphere to combat COVID-19. In this respect, it can be hypothesized that the coronavirus crisis has provided an opportunity to enhance Japan's human security policy and global health strategy.[15]

In retrospect, ever since the United Nations Development Program (UNDP) published their concept of human security in 1994, the Japanese government integrated it as one of the core pillars of its diplomatic policy.[16] Likewise, the Abe government facilitated Japan's human security diplomacy, and moreover, advocated its "global health strategy". For instance, a commentary by Prime Minister Abe entitled, "Japan's Strategy for Global Health Diplomacy: Why It Matters", was published on September 14, 2013, in the internationally renowned medical journal, *Lancet*. As an example of Japan's strategy on global health initiatives, Abe raised Japan's commitment to the fifth Tokyo International Conference on African Development (TICAD 5) held in June 2013, in which the premier called for the promotion of UHC and announced 500 million dollars of financial aid for the facilitation of a global health system.[17]

On December 12, 2015, Abe's commentary, "Japan's Vision for a Peaceful and Healthier World", was published in *Lancet* again.[18] Abe confirmed that "Japan has been a longstanding advocate of human security" and referred to the "2030 Agenda for Sustainable Development" adopted in the United Nations General Assembly in September 2015. Among the sustainable development goals (SDGs), the prime minister stressed the importance of UHC.[19] In the keynote speech at the TICAD 7 held on August 28, 2019, Abe stated that UHC is a quintessential example of "Brand Japan" and that Japan would work together with the "Global Alliance for Vaccines and Immunization" (Gavi, the Vaccine

[15] Clements, Kevin P. April 2020. "Confronting the Covid-19 Crisis: Danger and Opportunity". *Toda Peace Institute Director's Statement*. https://toda.org/assets/files/resources/policy-briefs/t-pb-71_kevin-clements_director-statement-on-covid-19.pdf.

[16] Edström, Bert. March 2011. "Japan and Human Security: The Derailing of a Foreign Policy Vision". *ISDP Asia Paper*. https://isdp.eu/content/uploads/images/stories/isdp-main-pdf/2011_edstrom_japan-and-human-security.pdf.

[17] Abe, Shinzo. September 14, 2013. "Japan's Strategy for Global Health Diplomacy: Why It Matters". *Lancet*. Vol. 382, No. 9896, pp. 915–916.

[18] Abe, Shinzo. December 12, 2015. "Japan's Vision for a Peaceful and Healthier World". *Lancet*. Vol. 386, No. 10011, pp. 2367–2369.

[19] Ibid.

Alliance).[20] Abe contended that Japan fully supports the efforts of the "World Bank's Pandemic Emergency Facility" and called for coordination between the WHO and the World Bank.[21] He moreover argued that the Japanese government would contribute to bringing together the expertise and resources for the global health system, including WHO, the World Bank, the Global Fund to Fight AIDS, Tuberculosis and Malaria, as well as Gavi.[22]

## Japan's Global Heath Policy and the COVID-19 Pandemic

Given Japan's human security diplomacy and global health strategy, it can be argued that the Abe government was expected to make more proactive contributions to combatting COVID-19 in the field of global health through promoting the development of coronavirus vaccines and the production of effective medicines. On March 28, 2020, Abe announced that the Japanese government would provide the "boldest ever" economic measures package of 56 trillion yen (518 billion dollars) to help reinvigorate the weakening Japanese economy affected by COVID-19.[23] At the same time, he stated that the government would approve the use of an anti-flu medicine, Avigan, as a treatment for the coronavirus-infected patients.[24]

Avigan (generic name: favipiravir), a product of Fujifilm Toyama Chemical Co., is purportedly able to shorten the recovery period of patients infected with COVID-19. Yet, Avigan has proven side effects for pregnant women, and it was reported that clinical trial of Avigan for COVID-19 patients would not be completed until the end of June

[20] Ministry of Foreign Affairs of Japan. August 28, 2019. "Keynote Address by Mr. Shinzo Abe, Prime Minister of Japan at the Opening Session of the Seventh Tokyo International Conference on African Development (TICAD 7)". https://www.mofa.go.jp/af/af1/page4e_001069.html.

[21] Ibid.

[22] Abe, Shinzo. December 12, 2015. "Japan's Vision for a Peaceful and Healthier World". *Lancet*. Vol. 386, No. 10011, pp. 2367–2369.

[23] Shibata, Nana. March 28, 2020. "Abe Says Japan Aims to Approve Avigan as Coronavirus Treatment". *Nikkei Asia*. https://asia.nikkei.com/Spotlight/Coronavirus/Abe-says-Japan-aims-to-approve-Avigan-as-coronavirus-treatment.

[24] Ibid.

2020.[25] Notably, the Abe government announced that Japan would offer Avigan to countries that wish to use it as a treatment of patients infected with COVID-19 free of charge. More than 30 countries subsequently requested Japan to provide Avigan. On March 31, 2020, Fujifilm Toyama Chemical Co. started the clinical tests, and on April 2, 2020, the German Health Ministry stated that they would purchase Avigan tablets from Japan.

On April 27, 2020, the Abe government submitted a supplementary budget of 25.69 trillion yen (240 billion dollars) as a package of emergency measures to mitigate Japan's economic damage and satisfy the basic needs of its citizens. This budget aimed to enable the government to provide 100,000 yen for all registered residents in Japan. Significantly, the extra budget was swiftly enacted on April 30 in order to accelerate the development of a coronavirus vaccine. The budget draft allocated to the domestic vaccine development was 10 billion yen, although it was estimated that 21.6 billion yen would be necessary for the international research and development of the vaccine in cooperation with international organizations.[26] For this reason, the Japanese government has been motivated to make more financial contributions to global health during the pandemic period.

## Japan's Contributions to Global Health Security

As discussed above, Japan has been active in contributing to global health as well as domestic public health, and the tendency became more conspicuous during the coronavirus pandemic period. Indeed, the WHO noted that "Japan has been a top ally of WHO during many emergencies, including the COVID-19 pandemic, the Ukraine crisis, natural disasters, and refugee crises worldwide" in the light of global health security.[27] It has been observed that the Shinzo Abe administration contributed to

[25] Bangkok Post. April 1, 2020. "Japan's Fujifilm Starts Avigan Trial to Treat Coronavirus". https://www.bangkokpost.com/world/1890935/japans-fujifilm-starts-avigan-trial-to-treat-coronavirus.

[26] Hasegawa, Tomoe. April 25, 2020. "Korona Wakuchin, Nihon ga Attoteki ni Deokureru Jijo (Reasons Why Japan Seriously Lags Behind in Developing Coronavirus Vaccines)". https://toyokeizai.net/articles/-/346439?page=4.

[27] World Health Organization (WHO). 2022. "Japan: A Champion for Health and Well-being at All Ages". https://www.who.int/about/funding/contributors/japan.

global health as pointed out by Haruka Sakamoto, Sarah Krull Abeis, and Satoshi Ezoe.[28] Based on Abe's contributions to global health security, Japan remained the fourth-largest donor to the Development Assistance Committee (DAC) of the Organization for Economic Cooperation and Development (OECD) in the field of global health during the coronavirus pandemic period (2021) as shown in the Fig. 1.1.[29]

Although Japan' ODA contribution was 26th among DAC donors in terms of its prioritization of global health in comparison to the size of the total ODA budget,[30] the Japanese government has consistently made financial contributions to the global health security especially in the COVID-19 pandemic. In 2021, Japan's global health spending was allocated for "COVID-19 control, health policy and administrative management, basic health infrastructure, medical services, infectious disease control, basic nutrition, reproductive health care, basic health care, health education, health personnel development, non-commutable

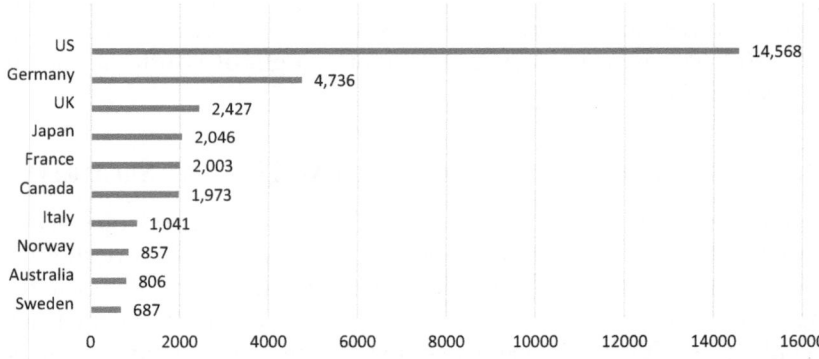

**Fig. 1.1** Top 10 countries in OECD members' contributions to global health in 2021 (*Note* Total ODA disbursements to the health sector [Unit = US million dollars])

---

[28] Sakamoto, Haruka, Sarah Krull Abeis, and Satoshi Ezoe. October 30, 2020. "Abe's Legacy: Japan's Contribution to Global Health". *BMJ Global Health*. https://blogs.bmj.com/bmjgh/2020/10/30/abes-legacy-japans-contribution-to-global-health/.

[29] Donor Tracker. July 20, 2023. "Japan / Global Health: ODA Spending". https://donortracker.org/donor_profiles/japan/globalhealth.

[30] Ibid.

diseases (NCDs) control, population policy and administrative management, medical education and training, malaria control, etc.".[31] This tendency has been enhanced by the successors of Abe, namely Yoshihide Suga and Fumio Kishida in the post-Abe administrations.[32] For this reason, it is important to examine Japan's global health policy in the post-Abe period including the Suga and Kishida administration, and this book aims to contextualize the development of Japan's global health strategy in the both pre- and post-COVID-19 world.

## CONCLUSION

The COVID-19 pandemic has in some way provided an opportunity for the reinvigoration of Japan's human security diplomacy and its role in the existing global health networks. As agreed between Abe and WHO Director-General Tedros Adhanom on March 30, 2020, Japan has been expected to contribute to the development of coronavirus vaccines and medicines in cooperation with other countries and international organizations.[33] Likewise, it has been argued that Japan's global health strategy to combat COVID-19 would be enhanced in collaboration with leading non-governmental organizations, such as the Gates Foundation as an international promotor of a global health system.

Through the international cooperation to combat COVID-19, Japan can make a more proactive contribution to promoting the establishment of a global health system in this human security crisis triggered by the coronavirus pandemic.[34] Thus, Japanese diplomacy for global health and human security has been strengthened in the coronavirus pandemic period, and Japan has taken concrete diplomatic and financial actions to fight against the COVID-19 pandemic as well as other infectious diseases

[31] Ibid.

[32] The Japanese Government. 2023. "Japan's International Cooperation for Global Health". *Highlighting Japan*. https://www.gov-online.go.jp/pdf/hlj/20230101/hlj202301_24-25_Japans_International_Cooperation_for_Global_Health.pdf.

[33] Ministry of Foreign Affairs of Japan. March 30, 2020. "Telephone Talk between Prime Minister ABE Shinzo and WHO Director-General Dr. Tedros Adhanom". https://www.mofa.go.jp/page1e_000277.html.

[34] Akimoto, Daisuke. May 6, 2020. "COVID-19 and Japan's Global Health Strategy: Developing Vaccines in a Human Security Crisis". *ISDP Voices*. https://isdp.eu/covid-19-japans-global-health-strategy/.

that threaten human security during the pandemic period. This book attempts to trace the development of Japan's global health policy in the pre-and post-COVID-19 pandemic. In addition, this research is based on my presentation, "Human Security Agenda in Japan's Global Health Strategy in the COVID-19 Pandemic Era", delivered at the Japan Association for Human Security Studies (JAHSS) held at Reitaku University on November 5, 2022.[35]

In the following chapters, this book will examine a variety of themes related to Japan and global health. Chapter 2 examines Japan, Gavi, and the COVID-19 Vaccines Global Access (COVAX) Facility for equal vaccine distribution in the COVID-19 pandemic. Chapter 3 analyzes the role of Japan in establishing and promoting the Global Fund to Fight AIDS, Tuberculosis and Malaria (Global Fund). Chapter 4 focuses on Japan's contribution to the Global Polio Eradication Initiative (GPEI) toward a "polio-free" world. Chapter 5 pays attention to Japan's commitments to the TICAD framework for the sake of global health and development in Africa. Chapter 6 contextualizes the development of Japan's policy on official development assistance (ODA) in terms of global health.

Chapter 7 highlights the role of the Japanese Business Leaders' Coalition for Global Health in the pandemic period. Chapter 8 investigates Japan's contributions to the Global Financing Facility for Women, Children and Adolescents (GFF) which is part of the World Bank and its significance for health and nutrition of women and children in the COVID-19 era. Chapter 9 sheds light on Japan's contributions to neglected tropical diseases (NTDs), while scrutinizing the role of the Global Health Innovative Technology Fund (GHIT Fund). Chapter 10 examines the emergence of Japan's global health strategy and its implications for the G7 Hiroshima Summit. Chapter 11 considers Japan's contributions to the Coalition for Epidemic Preparedness Innovations (CEPI) as pandemic preparedness and response for the next pandemic. Chapter 12 focuses on Japan and the role of the International Monetary Fund (IMF) and its "special drawing rights" (SDRs) during the coronavirus pandemic period. Finally, the concluding chapter summarizes the

---

[35] Daisuke Akimoto. November 5, 2022. "Human Security Agenda in Japan's Global Health Strategy in the COVID-19 Pandemic Era". Presentation at the Japan Association for Human Security Studies Annual Conference 2022. https://jahss2022.wixsite.com/mysite/day1.

findings of this research and discusses the emergence of a global health architecture in response to the COVID-19 pandemic and in preparation for pandemics in the future.

# CHAPTER 2

# Japan and Gavi: Its Global Health Diplomacy for the COVAX Facility

**Abstract** In terms of vaccine diplomacy, the Gavi, the Vaccine Alliance (Gavi), has made significant contributions toward immunizing the world's children against infectious diseases since its inception in 2000. From the perspective of Japan's global health diplomacy, its commitment to the "COVID-19 Vaccines Global Access" (COVAX) Facility has been of significance in the middle of the coronavirus pandemic. COVAX is a vaccines pillar of the Access to COVID-19 Tools Accelerator (ACT-A), and co-led by the Coalition for Epidemic Preparedness Innovations (CEPI), Gavi, the World Health Organization (WHO), and the United Nations Children's Fund (UNICEF). Given the significance of Gavi and the COVAX Facility as a facilitator and facility of global health, this chapter examines Japan's contributions to Gavi and the COVAX Facility.

**Keywords** Coronavirus (COVID-19) · COVAX Facility · Gavi · The Vaccine Alliance (Gavi) · Global health diplomacy · Japan

© The Author(s), under exclusive license to Springer Nature Singapore Pte Ltd. 2024
D. Akimoto, *Japan and Global Health*,
https://doi.org/10.1007/978-981-97-0972-4_2

# INTRODUCTION

In terms of vaccine diplomacy, the Gavi, the Vaccine Alliance (Gavi), has made significant contributions toward immunizing the world's children against infectious diseases since its inception in 2000.[1] From the perspective of Japan's global health diplomacy, its commitment to the "COVID-19 Vaccines Global Access" (COVAX) Facility has been of significance in the middle of the coronavirus pandemic.[2] COVAX is a vaccines pillar of the Access to COVID-19 Tools Accelerator (ACT-A), and co-led by the Coalition for Epidemic Preparedness Innovations (CEPI),[3] Gavi,[4] the World Health Organization (WHO), and the United Nations Children's Fund (UNICEF). As pointed out by Bill Gates during an interview one day after an international symposium, Global Health Action Japan, held in Tokyo on August 18, 2022, Japan was the first country that made a financial contribution to the COVAX Facility.[5]

It has been observed by researchers of global health and medical science that the COVAX Facility has made significant contributions to ensuing equitable access to "quality-assured vaccines" in the coronavirus pandemic period.[6] Notably, it has been analyzed that the COVAX Facility successfully incentivized high-income countries to participate in the vaccine redistribution system under which people in low-income countries can be vaccinated against the coronavirus.[7] Owing to its contribution to the equal distribution of coronavirus vaccines in the world including developing countries, the COVAX Facility was considered and

---

[1] Gavi. 2023. "About Our Alliance". https://www.gavi.org/our-alliance/about.

[2] World Health Organization (WHO). 2022. "COVAX". https://www.who.int/initiatives/act-accelerator/covax.

[3] CEPI. 2022. "COVAX: CEPI's Response to COVID-19". https://cepi.net/covax/.

[4] Gavi. 2022. "COVAX". https://www.gavi.org/covax-facility.

[5] Jiji. September 4, 2022. "Tojokoku no Iryokaizen wa Nihon no Rieki (Improvement of Medical Care in Developing Countries Is in Japan's Interest)". https://www.jiji.com/jc/v8?id=202209bill-gates-fukabori.

[6] Wakabayashi, Mami, Satoshi Ezoe, Makiko Yoneda, Yasushi Katsuma, and Hiroyasu Iso. 2021. "Global Landscape of the COVID-19 Vaccination Policy: Ensuring Equitable Access to Quality-Assured Vaccines". *GHM Open*. Vol. 2, No. 1, pp. 44–50.

[7] McAdams, David, Kaci Kennedy McDade, Osondu Ogbuoji, Matthew Johnson, Siddharth Dixit, and Gavin Yamey. 2020. "Incentivising Wealthy Nations to Participate in the COVID-19 Vaccine Global Access Facility (COVAX): A Game Theory Perspective". *BMJ Global Health*. Vol 5, No. 11, pp. 1–7.

selected as a nominee of the Nobel Peace Prize in 2021.[8] Given the significance of Gavi and the COVAX Facility as a facilitator and facility of global health, this chapter examines Japan's contributions to Gavi and the COVAX Facility.[9]

## Japan's Commitment to Gavi and the COVAX Facility

Japan has been one of the major donor countries to Gavi since 2011,[10] and made a continuous contribution to establishing and supporting the COVAX Facility as well. At the event of the G7 Ise-Shima Summit in 2016, the Japanese government announced a multi-year pledge to Gavi for the first time. In 2019, the Abe administration hosted Gavi's third replenishment conference as part of TICAD 7 in Yokohama.[11] During the coronavirus pandemic period, Japan pledged 300 million dollars to Gavi for 2021–2025 at the Global Vaccine Summit in June 2020, followed by another pledge of 200 million dollars to the COVAX Facility. Thus, the Japanese government made initial important diplomatic and financial commitments to Gavi as well as the COVAX Advance Market Commitment (AMC). Succeeding the legacy of Abe diplomacy, Prime Minister Yoshihide Suga pledged 800 million dollars at the COVAX AMC Summit held in June 2021.[12]

As pointed out by Kazuto Suzuki, a professor at the graduate school of public policy of the University of Tokyo, Japan's vaccine diplomacy is not that influenced by so-called "vaccine nationalism" which

---

[8] Japan Times. January 31, 2021. "Navalny, WHO and Thunberg among Nominees for Nobel Peace Prize". https://www.japantimes.co.jp/news/2021/01/31/world/nobel-peace-prize-nominees/.

[9] This chapter is based on my earlier research on Japan's contributions to the COVAX Facility. See Akimoto, Daisuke. July 12, 2022. "Japan's Global Health Diplomacy and the COVAX Facility". *ISDP Voices*. https://www.isdp.eu/japans-global-health-diplomacy-and-the-covax-facility/.

[10] National Institute of Infectious Diseases. 2017. *IASR*. Vol. 38, No. 3 (No. 445), March 2017, pp. 67–68. https://www.niid.go.jp/niid/ja/vaccine-j/1685-idsc/iasr-out/7146-445f01.html.

[11] Gavi. 2023. "Donor Profiles: Japan (as of June 30, 2023)". https://www.gavi.org/investing-gavi/funding/donor-profiles/japan.

[12] Ibid.

causes monopolization of vaccines in a country.[13] This is because the Japanese government has supported the COVAX Facility based on its "human security as a guiding principle for global health",[14] which can be regarded as international cooperation. Hence, the Japanese government contributed to the establishment of the COVAX Facility and has continued to strengthen the global vaccine distribution system during the pandemic period.

On April 8, 2022, the Gavi COVAX AMC Summit was held under the leadership of co-hosts, the Governments of Germany (G7 Presidency), Ghana, Indonesia (G20 Presidency), Senegal (African Union Chair), as well as the Gavi, the Vaccine Alliance.[15] The summit was aimed to facilitate equitable access to safe, effective, and quality-assured coronavirus vaccines in both developed and developing countries in response to the COVID-19 pandemic. At the summit, Prime Minister Fumio Kishida stated that there is a "vaccine equity gap" in the world, and that Japan had already donated more than 43 million doses of vaccines to countries in need.[16]

Kishida pledged that Japan would contribute up to 500 million dollars to COVAX on top of the previous contribution of billion dollars which was already disbursed. In his video message, Kishida stated that "The key to truly overcoming this pandemic is to ensure equitable access to vaccines in every country and region of the world so that no one's health is left behind".[17] As shown in Fig. 2.1, the Japanese government has made considerable financial contributions to Gavi since its inception. During the period from 2011 to 2015, Japan made direct contributions of 53.7 million dollars to Gavi. From 2016 to 2020, Japan donated 94.7 million

---

[13] Suzuki, Kazuto. February 26, 2021. "Japan's Vaccine Strategy". *The Diplomat*. https://thediplomat.com/2021/02/japans-vaccine-strategy/.

[14] Shibuya, Kenji, Chorh Chuan Tan, Asaph Young Chun, and Gabriel M. Leung. 2022. "Global Human Security in the Post-COVID-19 Era: The Rising Role of East Asia". *PLOS Medicine*. Vol. 19, No. 7, pp. 1–11.

[15] Gavi. April 8, 2022. "Break COVID Now". https://www.gavi.org/sites/default/files/covid/covax/Gavi-Break-COVID-Now-Summit-2022-Chairs-Summary.pdf.

[16] Ministry of Foreign Affairs of Japan. 2022. "Gavi COVAX AMC Summit 2022 Statement by H.E. Fumio Kishida, Prime Minister of Japan". https://www.mofa.go.jp/files/100329713.pdf.

[17] Kyodo News. April 8, 2022. "Japan PM Pledges $500 Mil. for Global Vaccine-sharing Efforts". https://english.kyodonews.net/news/2022/04/7e83ee83ccab-japan-pm-pledges-500-mil-to-global-far-vaccine-sharing-efforts.html.

dollars to Gavi. These two figures are low compared to the pandemic period, because the COVAX Facility was not established during the period. After the establishment of the COVAX Facility however, Japan's financial contributions amounted to 140 million dollars as direct contribution, and as much as 1500 million dollars to the COVAX AMC from 2021 to 2025. Although Japan has not pledged its financial contributions to Gavi during the period from 2026 to 2037 yet, these figures indicate that Japan's contributions to Gavi have been substantial, and it can be inferred that the country would continue its financial contributions to Gavi in the foreseeable future.[18]

In total, Japan's financial contributions to Gavi amounted to as much as 1540.1 million dollars as of June 30, 2023. Specifically, Japan donated 100.1 million dollars as direct funding to Gavi, whereas it contributed 1440 million dollars to the COVAX AMC so far. These figures suggest that the Japanese government from the Abe administration to the Kishida administration has actively supported Gavi in both pre-and post-pandemic

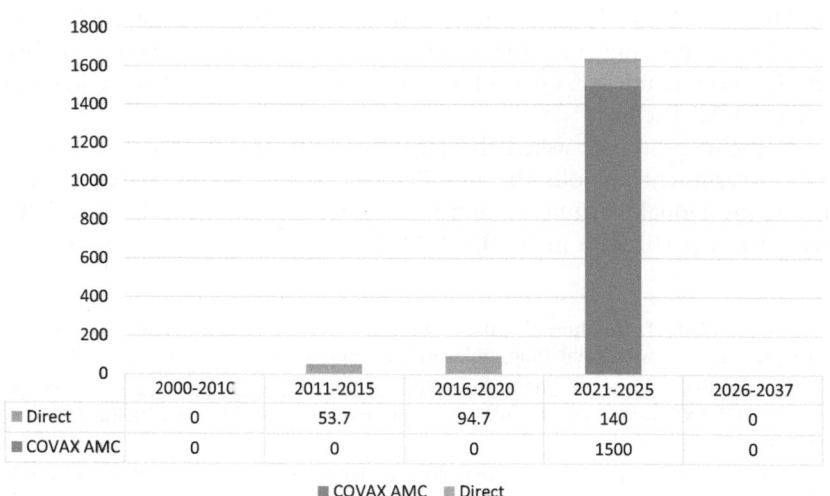

| | 2000-2010 | 2011-2015 | 2016-2020 | 2021-2025 | 2026-2037 |
|---|---|---|---|---|---|
| ■ Direct | 0 | 53.7 | 94.7 | 140 | 0 |
| ■ COVAX AMC | 0 | 0 | 0 | 1500 | 0 |

■ COVAX AMC  ■ Direct

**Fig. 2.1** Japan's contributions and Pledges to Gavi Over Time (*Note* Unit = US million dollars)

[18] Gavi. 2023. "Donor Profiles: Japan (as of June 30, 2023)". https://www.gavi.org/investing-gavi/funding/donor-profiles/japan.

periods. In a way, it is fair to argue that Japan's global health diplomacy toward the COVAX Facility is consistent with Prime Minister Kishida's "new capitalism" that values a redistribution of wealth and a virtuous cycle of growth on a global scale.[19]

## JAPAN'S ENTRY INTO THE COVAX FACILITY: DOMESTIC AND EXTERNAL ASPECTS

Importantly, Japan became one of the first developed countries to participate in the COVAX Facility. On August 18, 2020, Komeito, a junior coalition partner of the Liberal Democratic Party (LDP), officially requested that the Japanese government should consider and decide on Japan's early participation in the COVAX Facility. On August 27, Komeito's Chief Representative Natsuo Yamaguchi reconfirmed the party's request in order to secure necessary vaccines for Japan and provide vaccines for developing countries in need.[20] On August 31, the Japanese government expressed its willingness to participate in the COVAX Facility, and took a cabinet decision on September 15, 2020, to spend 17.2 billion yen for Japan's entry into the facility.[21] Meanwhile, Seth Berkley as CEO of Gavi commended Komeito for its role in facilitating Japan's entry into the COVAX Facility.[22]

Komeito moreover asked the Japanese government to encourage the US government to join the multilateral vaccine supply system. Previously, the Donald Trump administration declared that the United States would not participate in the COVAX Facility,[23] whereas China decided

[19] NHK World Japan. June 7, 2022. "Kishida's 'New Capitalism' Shifts Emphasis to Growth". https://www3.nhk.or.jp/nhkworld/en/news/videos/20220607211259765/.

[20] Sankei Biz. August 27, 2020. "Komeito Leader Yamaguchi Urges Japan's Participation in COVAX". https://www.sankeibiz.jp/macro/news/200827/mca2008271424018-n1.htm.

[21] Ministry of Health, Labour and Welfare of Japan. September 15, 2020. "Overview of Press Interview by Minister Kato". https://www.mhlw.go.jp/stf/kaiken/daijin/0000194708_00276.html.

[22] Komeito. October 17, 2020. "Gavi CEO Thanks Komeito for COVAX Support". https://www.komei.or.jp/komeinews/p124659/.

[23] Friedman, Eric A., Lawrence O. Gostin, Matthew M. Kavanagh, John T. Monahan, and Harold Hongju Koh. September 15, 2020. "Joining COVAX Could Save American Lives". *Foreign Policy*. https://foreignpolicy.com/2020/09/15/covax-vaccine-covid-19-trump-save-lives-equitable-distribution/.

to join the COVAX program backed by the WHO.[24] During the Cabinet Committee of the Upper House on October 8, 2020, Mitsuo Takahashi, a lawmaker of Komeito, stated that Tokyo would need to encourage Washington to join the COVAX system regardless of the result of the presidential election scheduled the following month.[25] On hearing this, a government official responded that Japan would continue to explain the importance of the COVAX Facility to many countries, including the United States.[26]

Likewise, Yuzuru Takeuchi of Komeito argued in the Budget Committee of the Lower House on November 2, 2020 that the Japanese government should encourage both the United States and Russia to join the COVAX Facility.[27] In response, Prime Minister Yoshihide Suga promised that Japan would continue to call on the United States to join the system.[28] Although the role of the Japanese government in facilitating the increase of member-states of the COVAX Facility is not measurable, President Joe Biden announced on January 21, 2021, that the United States would join the multilateral vaccine distribution system.[29] As a result of the strong urging by Komeito as a ruling party, Japan became one of the first developed countries to join the COVAX Facility and kept on urging Washington to participate in COVAX system.

[24] Qian, Colin and Stephanie Nebehay. October 9, 2020. "China Joins WHO-Backed Vaccine Programme COVAX Rejected by Trump". *Reuters*. https://jp.reuters.com/article/us-health-coronavirus-china-covax/china-joins-who-backed-vaccine-programme-covax-rejected-by-trump-idUSKBN26U027.

[25] National Diet Library. October 8, 2020. "Proceedings of the 202nd Diet Session. Cabinet Committee, the House of Councillors". https://kokkai.ndl.go.jp/#/detail?minId=120214889X00120201008&spkNum=97&single.
https://kokkai.ndl.go.jp/#/detail?minId=120214889X00120201008&spkNum=98&single.

[26] Ibid.

[27] National Diet Library. November 2, 2020. "Proceedings of the 202nd Diet Session. Budget Committee, the House of Representatives". https://kokkai.ndl.go.jp/#/detail?minId=120305261X00220201102&spkNum=128&single.
https://kokkai.ndl.go.jp/txt/120305261X00220201102/129.

[28] Ibid.

[29] Rouw, Anna, Jennifer Kates, Josh Michaud, and Adam Wexler. February 18, 2021. "COVAX and the United States". KFF. https://www.kff.org/coronavirus-covid-19/issue-brief/covax-and-the-united-states/.

Although Komeito made important initial contributions and continuous commitments to the COVAX Facility, it is not the only political party that supports the facility. In fact, Diet members of other political parties also started supporting the multilateral coronavirus vaccine redistribution system. On August 20, 2020, Akiko Honda of the LDP pointed out the importance of the COVAX Facility during the Committee on Health, Labour and Welfare in the House of Councillors. With her background as a chemist, Honda also argued that it would be important for the government to support pharmaceutical companies during the coronavirus pandemic.[30]

On June 11, 2021, Yuriko Yamakawa from the Constitutional Democratic Party of Japan (Rikken Minshuto) asked a question about coronavirus vaccines made by Astra Zeneca and the COVAX Facility to Minister of Health, Labour and Welfare Norihisa Tamura. Minister Tamura replied that the coronavirus vaccines of Astra Zeneca were approved by the Ministry of Health, Labour and Welfare.[31] On March 23, 2022, Kohei Otsuka from the Democratic Party For the People (Kokumin Minshuto) pointed out that the COVAX Facility supports not only vaccine distribution but development of the vaccines as well. Otsuka therefore argued that Japan also should be able to make a contribution to the development of vaccines through the COVAX Facility. A government official replied that the Japanese government would like to support Japanese companies so that they could be subsidized by CEPI in the field of vaccine development, etc.[32] Indeed, CEPI as part of the COVAX Facility has been a major contributor to the development of vaccines in preparation for and in response to pandemics.

On May 20, 2022, Hirobumi Niki from Yushi no Kai pointed out that Japan's financial contributions to the COVAX Facility accounted for about 10 percent of the total donation and that many coronavirus

[30] National Diet Library. August 20, 2020. "Proceedings of the 201st Diet Session. Committee on Health, Labour and Welfare, the House of Councillors". https://kokkai.ndl.go.jp/#/detail?minId=120114260X00220200820&spkNum=16&current=78.

[31] National Diet Library. June 11, 2021. "Proceedings of the 204th Diet Session. Committee on Health, Labour and Welfare, the House of Representatives". https://kokkai.ndl.go.jp/#/detail?minId=120404260X02720210611&spkNum=158&current=30.

[32] National Diet Library. March 23, 2022. "Proceedings of the 208th Diet Session. Special Committee on the Official Development Assistance, etc. and Okinawa and Northern Territories, the House of Councillors". https://kokkai.ndl.go.jp/#/detail?minId=120815359X00420220323&spkNum=56&current=15.

vaccines ended up with passing the expiration date. In response, Taro Honda as Vice-Minister for the Ministry of Foreign Affairs explained that the Japanese government supported the development of so-called "cold-chain" from airport to vaccination places as last-one-mile support.[33]

On October 13, 2022, Atsushi Suzuki of the Democratic Party For the People discussed that North Korea used to reject receiving coronavirus vaccines by the COVAX Facility, but it finally started vaccination in late August of the year.[34] On March 16, 2023, Mitsuko Ishii of Japan Innovation Party (Ishin) asked the importance of the COVAX Facility. In response, a government official explained that the facility had provided 1.9 billion doses of COVID-19 vaccines around the world and emphasized the fact that 74 percent of coronavirus vaccines was provided through the COVAX Facility.[35] Thus, it is no exaggeration to argue that there exists a multipartisan support for Gavi and the COVAX Facility in Japan.

## Japan's Direct and Indirect Vaccine Donations and the FOIP Vision

Why has Japan been eager to make financial contributions to the COVAX Facility? For one thing, human security is a core diplomatic pillar, but at the same time, it is also related to its Free and Open Indo-Pacific (FOIP) vision. On June 2, 2021, the Japanese government under the leadership of Prime Minister Yoshihide Suga pledged additional 800 million dollars to the COVAX Facility during an online summit meeting. Suga also promised that Japan would provide 30 million domestically produced doses in the future. At the meeting, Suga stated that "We must not allow a country's specific situation or economic power to determine its access to

---

[33] National Diet Library. May 20, 2022. "Proceedings of the 208th Diet Session. Health, Labour and Welfare Committee, the House of Representatives". https://kokkai.ndl.go.jp/#/detail?minId=120804260X02120220520&spkNum=154&current=8.

[34] National Diet Library. October 13, 2022. "Proceeding of the 210th Diet Session. Foreign Affairs Committee, the House of Representatives". https://kokkai.ndl.go.jp/#/detail?minId=121005365X00120221013&spkNum=108&current=5.

[35] National Diet Library. March 16, 2023. "Proceeding of the 211th Diet Session. Special Committee on the Official Development Assistance etc. and Okinawa and Northern Territories, the House of Councillors". https://kokkai.ndl.go.jp/#/detail?minId=121115359X00320230316&spkNum=78&current=1.

vaccines… Japan fully supports efforts to ensure equitable access to safe and effective vaccines for as many people as possible".[36] Given the significance of the FOIP vision, it can be argued that Japan strengthened its vaccination support for developing countries to counter Beijing's vaccine diplomacy, fearing political influence over recipient nations.[37] Moreover, the Japanese government has reinforced its strategic partnership with the so-called Quad countries, such as Australia, India, and the United States. The Quad vaccine partnership represents Japan's strategic commitment to the global health system.[38]

According to a government document entitled "Japan's COVID-19 Vaccine-Related Support" announced by the Ministry of Foreign Affairs, Japan in May 2022, the Japanese government had already disbursed 1 billion dollars to AMC of COVAX Facility, carried out so-called "last one mile" support for capacity building of medical experts and cold chain system in 77 countries and areas with 18 billion dollars through the Japan International Cooperation Agency (JICA) and the UNICEF, and conducted direct and indirect donations of coronavirus vaccines for approximately 44 million doses in total so far.[39] Japan's direct donations of COVID-19 vaccines amounted to 24.65 million doses, and vaccine recipient countries include Taiwan (4.2 million doses), Vietnam (7.35 million doses), Indonesia (6.88 million doses), Malaysia (1 million doses), the Philippines (3.08 million doses), Thailand (2.04 million doses), and Brunei (0.1 million doses)—all of which are strategically important countries in the Indo-Pacific area.

As for indirect donations through the COVAX Facility, Japan has made financial contributions to 19.38 million doses of COVID-19 vaccines. Recipient countries on the list in the government document are Cambodia (1.32 million doses), Laos (0.94 million doses), East Timor (0.17 million doses), Bangladesh (4.55 million doses), Maldives (0.11

---

[36] Japan Times. June 3, 2021. "Japan Pledges $800 Million for Global COVID-19 Vaccination Effort". https://www.japantimes.co.jp/news/2021/06/03/national/science-health/japan-covax-donation/.

[37] Ibid.

[38] Ministry of Foreign Affairs of Japan. April 12, 2022. "Vaccine Donation to Cambodia by Japan-Australia-India-U.S. (Quad)". https://www.mofa.go.jp/press/release/press1e_0 00283.html.

[39] Ministry of Foreign Affairs of Japan. May 2022. "Japan's COVID-19 Vaccine-Related Support". https://www.mofa.go.jp/files/100226669.pdf.

million doses), Tajikistan (0.5 million doses), Uzbekistan (0.2 million doses), Nepal (1.61 million doses), Sri Lanka (1.46 million doses), Pacific Island Countries (0.34 million doses), Nicaragua (0.5 million doses), Iran (4.31 million doses), Syria (0.15 million doses), Egypt (0.7 million doses), Malawi (0.68 million doses), Nigeria (0.86 million doses), Cameroon (0.07 million doses), Ghana (0.31 million doses), Senegal (0.3 million doses), Kenya (0.2 million doses), and Sierra Leone (0.1 million doses).[40] As these figures indicate, the Japanese government has made continuous contributions to the fair redistribution of coronavirus vaccines. Thus, it is critical to note that Japan has supported many countries of the Indo-Pacific region, and therefore, it is possible to analyze that Tokyo's vaccine diplomacy has been fundamentally influenced not only by its human security diplomacy but also by its FOIP vision in the era of the Indo-Pacific geopolitics.

## Conclusion

This chapter has investigated Japan's financial and diplomatic contributions to Gavi as well as the COVAX Facility during the coronavirus pandemic. It contextualized Japan's incremental and continuous contributions to Gavi by tracing the pledged amount of direct contribution and the COVAX AMC. It was highlighted that Japan's total financial contributions to Gavi amounted to 1540.1 million dollars as of June 30, 2023. This chapter moreover clarified that Japan's entry into the COVAX Facility was facilitated by Komeito and later supported by other political parties. The multipartisan support for the multilateral vaccine distribution system enabled Japan to make proactive contributions to direct and indirect vaccine donations to developing countries. Although Japan's diplomatic contributions to the developing countries have been based on the national interests, it contributed to strengthening the global health system based on the human security concept as well as international cooperation as well.

Some COVID-19 vaccines under license contracts with Astra Zeneca or Novavax have been domestically developed in Japan, and they have been supplied to other countries as part of the government's direct

[40] Ibid.

vaccine donation program.[41] This could be regarded as Japan's international cooperation and global health diplomacy during the coronavirus pandemic. Nevertheless, there exists no domestically developed or original vaccines in Japan so far. Regarding this matter, Isao Teshirogi, President and CEO of Shionogi, representing the Federation of Pharmaceutical Manufacturers' Associations of JAPAN, pointed out that Japan had made financial contributions to the COVAX Facility, but the country was not able to make direct contributions to the facility in terms of the development of purely domestically developed COVID-19 vaccines. Teshirogi argued that domestic development of vaccines as a measure against the pandemic was a critical factor for Japan's national security.[42]

To contribute to the COVAX Facility in terms of vaccine development as well as financial contribution, it is imperative for the Kishida government to reinforce national pharmaceutical companies. It does not mean, however, that Japanese people should depend only on domestically produced vaccines, because such a measure might lead to vaccine nationalism. Still, it is important for Japanese pharmaceutical companies to develop and produce original vaccines, because it could be meaningful to the enhancement of the global health system as well as to current and future Japanese global health diplomacy in the pandemic and post-pandemic periods. In essence, although the COVAX Facility terminated its activities on December 31, 2023,[43] Japan's global health diplomacy toward Gavi has been in line with Prime Minister Kishida's new capitalism for redistribution of vaccines as opposed to vaccine nationalism.

[41] Ministry of Health, Labour and Welfare of Japan. June 4, 2021. "International Cooperation through Domestically Produced Coronavirus Vaccines". https://www.mhlw.go.jp/stf/newpage_19070.html. See also, Takeda. April 19, 2022. "Takeda Announces Approval of Nuvaxovid® COVID-19 Vaccine for Primary and Booster Immunization in Japan". https://www.takeda.com/newsroom/newsreleases/2022/takeda-announces-approval-of-nuvaxovid-covid-19-vaccine-for-primary-and-booster-immunization-in-japan/.

[42] Teshirogi, Isao. April 16, 2021. "Significance of Purely Domestically Developed COVID-19 Vaccines in Light of National Security". Federation of Pharmaceutical Manufacturers' Associations of JAPAN (FPMAJ). https://www.kantei.go.jp/jp/singi/kenkou iryou/iyakuhin/dai4/siryou1-2.pdf.

[43] World Health Organization (WHO). December 19, 2023. "COVID-19 Vaccinations Shift to Regular Immunization as COVAX Draws to a Close". https://www.who.int/news/item/19-12-2023-covid-19-vaccinations-shift-to-regular-immunization-as-covax-draws-to-a-close.

# CHAPTER 3

# Japan and the Global Fund to Fight AIDS, Tuberculosis and Malaria

**Abstract** During the coronavirus (COVID-19) pandemic, Japan has made diplomatic efforts for the enhancement of the global health system in conjunction with the Global Fund to Fight AIDS, Tuberculosis and Malaria (Global Fund). The Global Fund was established in January 2002 based on a statement by Japanese Prime Minister Yoshiro Mori who mentioned the importance of establishing new partnerships and international cooperation to fight against infectious diseases at the Kyushu-Okinawa G8 Summit in 2000. Since then, Japan has made diplomatic contributions to the development of the Global Fund. Given the significance of the Global Fund to the global health system, this chapter examines Japan's contributions to the Global Fund since its inception to the present including the COVID-19 pandemic period.

**Keywords** Coronavirus (COVID-19) · Global Fund to Fight AIDS · Tuberculosis and Malaria (Global Fund) · HIV/AIDS · Japan · Malaria · Tuberculosis

## Introduction

During the COVID-19 pandemic, Japan has made diplomatic efforts for the enhancement of the global health system in conjunction with the Global Fund to Fight AIDS, Tuberculosis and Malaria (Global Fund).[1] On April 21, 2022, Peter Sands, Executive Director of the Global Fund paid a courtesy visit to Japanese Foreign Minister Yoshimasa Hayashi.[2] Hayashi praised the role of the Global Fund for attempting to combat the three major infectious diseases in the middle of the coronavirus pandemic. Director Sands appreciated Japan's continuous contributions to the Global Fund and reported the status quo of infectious diseases in Ukraine after the outbreak of the Russia-Ukraine conflict. Both Hayashi and Sands agreed to continue further cooperation for achieving universal health coverage (UHC) and improving the global health system to prevent and prepare for future pandemics.

The Global Fund was established in January 2002 based on a statement by Japanese Prime Minister Yoshiro Mori who mentioned the importance of establishing "new partnerships" and international cooperation to fight against infectious diseases at the Kyushu-Okinawa G8 Summit in 2000.[3] Notably, it was announced in the G8 Communique Okinawa 2000 that the Group of Eight (G8) would strengthen its partnership with other governments and the World Health Organization (WHO) to reduce the number of HIV/AIDS-infected young people by 25 percent, deaths by tuberculosis and prevalence of the disease by 50 percent, and the burden of disease associated with malaria by 50 percent, by 2010.[4]

In June 2005, Prime Minister Junichiro Koizumi pledged 500 million dollars to the Global Fund and reiterated 5 billion dollars pledge over five years as Japan's official development assistance (ODA) for health

---

[1] The Global Fund. 2022. "The Global Fund to Fight AIDS, Tuberculosis and Malaria". https://www.theglobalfund.org/en/.

[2] Ministry of Foreign Affairs of Japan. April 21, 2022. "Courtesy Call on Foreign Minister Hayashi Yoshimasa by Mr. Peter Sands, Executive Director of the Global Fund". https://www.mofa.go.jp/press/release/press1e_000285.html.

[3] Mori, Yoshiro. June 5, 2000. "Address by Prime Minister Yoshiro Mori at the Discussion Group on the Kyushu-Okinawa Summit, Okinawa Summit". *"The World and Japan"* *Database*. https://worldjpn.grips.ac.jp/documents/texts/summit/20000605.S1E.html.

[4] Ministry of Foreign Affairs of Japan. July 23, 2000. "G8 Communique Okinawa 2000". https://www.mofa.go.jp/policy/economy/summit/2000/documents/communique.html.

and development.[5] Koizumi said that these decisions had been made based on "human security" as one of core pillars of Japanese diplomacy.[6] In a symposium, "From Okinawa to Toyako: Dealing with Communicable Diseases as Global Human Security Threats" held on May 23, 2008, Prime Minister Yasuo Fukuda recalled the role of the Kyushu-Okinawa Summit during which the establishment of the Global Fund was proposed, and stated that Japan as a "peace fostering nation" should make contributions to international health cooperation for combating the three major infectious diseases.[7]

As a result of the G8 Hokkaido-Toyako Summit held in July 2008, the Task Force on Global Action for Health System Strengthening submitted a report as policy recommendations to the G8.[8] The task force was composed of global health policy experts, including Keizo Takemi as a Diet member of the Upper House, future Minister of Health, Labour and Welfare, former Tokai University Professor, and a research fellow at Harvard School of Public Health.[9] Thus, Japan made a diplomatic contribution to the establishment and the development of the Global Fund. Given the significance of the Global Fund to the global health system,

[5] Ministry of Foreign Affairs of Japan. June 30, 2005. "Prime Minister Koizumi Pledges 'US$ 500 Million for the Coming Years' to the Global Fund, Reiterates US$ 5 Billion Pledge over 5 Years for Health in ODA". https://www.mofa.go.jp/announce/announce/2005/6/0630.html.

[6] Ministry of Foreign Affairs of Japan. June 30, 2005. "Address by Prime Minister Junichiro Koizumi at the Commemorative Symposium on the Fifth Anniversary of the Kyusyu-Okinawa Summit: East Asian Regional Response to HIV/AIDS, Tuberculosis and Malaria". https://www.mofa.go.jp/policy/health_c/gfatm/address0506.html.

[7] Ministry of Foreign Affairs of Japan. May 23, 2008. Opening Remarks by H.E. Mr. Yasuo Fukuda, Prime Minister of Japan on the Occasion of "From Okinawa to Toyako: Dealing with Communicable Diseases as Global Human Security Threats". https://www.mofa.go.jp/policy/health_c/remark0805.html.

[8] Japan Center for International Exchange (JCIE). 2009. "G8 Hokkaido Toyako Summit Follow-Up Global Action for Health System Strengthening Policy Recommendations to the G8 (by Task Force on Global Action for Health System Strengthening)". https://www.jcie.org/wp-content/uploads/2021/07/takemi-full.pdf.

[9] Holmes, David. August 30, 2011. "Keizo Takemi: A Catalytic Charisma". *Lancet*. Vol. 378, No. 9796, p. 1065.

this chapter examines Japan's contributions to the Global Fund since its inception to the present.[10]

## Multi-partisan Support for Japan's Financial Contributions to the Global Fund

During the administration by the Democratic Party of Japan (DPJ), the Japanese government continued its contribution to the Global Fund. State Secretary for Foreign Affairs Yutaka Banno of the Naoto Kan administration pledged 800 million dollars at the Third Voluntary Replenishment Conference of the Global Fund held on October 5, 2010, in New York. On June 3, 2011, Banno stated that although Japan had suffered from the Great East Japan Earthquake, its policy on international cooperation including contribution to the Global Fund would not be changed.[11] Banno's remarks indicate that Japan's policy on the Global Fund had been consistent during the DPJ administration, even after the nationwide disasters in 2011.

After the Liberal Democratic Party (LDP) and Komeito came back to power in 2012, the LDP-Komeito coalition government resumed the contributions to the Global Fund. On March 12, 2013, Vice-Foreign Minister Masaji Matsuyama met Mark Dybul, Executive Director of the Global Fund, and encouraged him to participate in the Fifth Tokyo International Conference on African Development (TICAD 5). In response, Executive Director Dybul stated that he would attend the conference and cooperate with Japan in the field of global health.[12] On December 3, 2013, Parliamentary Vice-Minister for Foreign Affairs Seiji Kihara as a special envoy of Prime Minister Shinzo Abe delivered a speech at the Fourth Voluntary Replenishment Conference of the Global Fund. Kihara

[10] This chapter is based on my earlier research on Japan and the Global Fund. See, Akimoto, Daisuke. June 2, 2022. "Japan's Diplomatic Commitment to the Global Fund". *ISDP Voices*. https://www.isdp.eu/japan-committed-to-support-global-fund/.

[11] Ministry of Foreign Affairs of Japan. October 5, 2010. "Speech by State Secretary for Foreign Affairs Yutaka BANNO at the Third Voluntary Replenishment Conference of the Global Fund to Fight AIDS, Tuberculosis and Malaria". https://www.mofa.go.jp/announce/svm/speech101006.html.

[12] Ministry of Foreign Affairs of Japan. March 12, 2013. "Courtesy Call on Vice-Foreign Minister Masaji Matsuyama by Mr. Mark Dybul, Executive Director of the Global Fund". https://www.mofa.go.jp/mofaj/annai/honsho/fuku/matsuyama/wf_130312.html.

stressed the importance of human security and the realization of UHC, and pledged 800 million dollars in the coming years.[13]

On December 17, 2015, Foreign Minister Fumio Kishida made a speech at the Fifth Replenishment Preparatory Meeting of the Global Fund, and expressed Japan's further support for the Global Fund based on human security concept, while referring to the significance of the 2000 Kyushu-Okinawa Summit and Japan's G7 presidency in 2016.[14] During the Sixth Voluntary Replenishment Conference held on October 9–10, 2016, State Minister for Foreign Affairs Keisuke Suzuki mentioned that Japan would host the G20 Osaka Summit and TICAD 7 in 2016, and pledged 840 million dollars to the Global Fund, a 5 percent increase compared to the amount pledged in the previous replenishment conference.[15] Thus, it can be observed that Kishida as foreign minister was active in facilitating Japan's global health diplomacy for the Global Fund in the Abe administration.

On March 25, 2021, the Parliamentary Group to End Malaria by 2030 in Japan was established by bipartisan Diet members. Yasuhisa Shiozaki, a member of the House of Representatives of the LDP, became a chair of the parliamentary group. As an active facilitator of malaria eradication, Malaria No More Japan (MNMJ) welcomed the establishment of the parliamentary group as the "face of the legislature" in the global malaria eradication movement.[16] On July 19, 2022, a "Request for Malaria Control along with the Promotion of Irrigated Rice Cultivation in Sub-Saharan Africa" was submitted by MNMJ to Takeaki Matsumoto

[13] Ministry of Foreign Affairs of Japan. December 3, 2013. "Speech by Parliamentary Vice-Minister for Foreign Affairs Seiji KIHARA at the Fourth Voluntary Replenishment Conference of the Global Fund to Fight AIDS, Tuberculosis and Malaria". https://www.mofa.go.jp/mofaj/files/000023126.pdf.

[14] Ministry of Foreign Affairs of Japan. December 17, 2015. "Remarks by Foreign Minister Kishida at the 5th Replenishment Preparatory Meeting of the Global Fund. (December 17, 2015 at Tokyo Prince Hotel)". https://www.mofa.go.jp/ic/ghp/page24e_000124.html.

[15] Ministry of Foreign Affairs of Japan. October 9–10, 2016. "Speech by State Minister for Foreign Affairs of Japan, Mr. SUZUKI Keisuke". https://www.mofa.go.jp/mofaj/files/000526525.pdf.

[16] Malaria No More Japan. March 26, 2021. "Welcome to the Establishment of the Parliamentary Group to End Malaria by 2030 in Japan". https://malarianomore.jp/wp_core/wp-content/uploads/2021/03/Parliamentary-Group-Launch_pressrelease_0326_final.pdf.

as a chair of the parliamentary group.[17] The example of the parliamentary group shows Japan's willingness to make political and financial contributions to the Global Fund.

As a matter of fact, the Japanese government has made consistent contributions to the Global Fund as shown in Fig. 3.1.[18] According to the source by the Global Fund, Japan was the fifth largest public donor to the Global Fund, donating a total of 4.57 billion dollars as of the end of 2022.[19] Notably, Japan's pledge and the amount of actual donation have been accorded since 2001 to the present. Even during the 2008 Global Financial Crisis and the 2011 Great East Japan Earthquake, the Japanese government continued the pledges and made the pledged contributions to the Global Fund. This indicates that Japan has kept its promise as opposed to some other public donors that did not fulfill their pledges. In this sense, it can be argued that Japan has been expected to contribute the rest of the pledged amount to the Global Fund by the end of 2025.

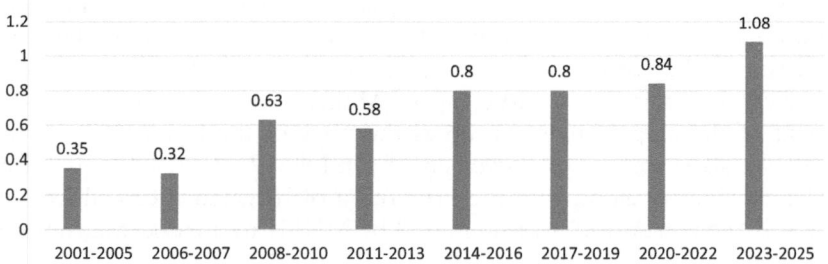

**Fig. 3.1** Japan's donations to the Global Fund by replenishment (*Note* Source by the Global Fund as of the end of 2022 [Unit = US billion dollars])

[17] Malaria No More Japan. July 19, 2022. "Request for Malaria Control along with the Promotion of Irrigated Rice Cultivation in Sub-Saharan Africa". https://malarianomore.jp/wp_core/wp-content/uploads/2022/07/20220719policyrecommendation_Eng.pdf.

[18] The Global Fund. 2023. "Government and Public Donors: Japan". https://www.theglobalfund.org/en/government/profiles/japan/; and Ministry of Finance Japan. 2022. "Sokatsu Chosahyo: The Global Fund (Summary Survey on the Global Fund)". https://www.mof.go.jp/policy/budget/topics/budget_execution_audit/fy2022/sy0407/7.pdf.

[19] The Global Fund. 2023. "Government and Public Donors: Japan". https://www.theglobalfund.org/en/government/profiles/japan/.

## Infectious Diseases and Humanitarian Crisis in War-Torn Ukraine

During the Kishida administration, the Japanese government has continued to make diplomatic efforts for the Global Fund. On February 24, 2022, Osamu Kunii as a Management Executive Committee member of the Global Fund paid a courtesy visit to Vice-Foreign Minister Takako Suzuki.[20] Both Suzuki and Kunii agreed that it is important to foster experts and activists who can contribute to the field of global health.[21] As a matter of fact, Kunii has been actively committed to advocacy activities to Japanese lawmakers to promote the vision and mission of the Global Fund.[22] Furthermore, Takeshi Akahori, Ambassador, Director-General for Global Issues of the Foreign Ministry, visited Geneva and had talks with Executive Director Peter Sands on April 8, 2022. Both Sands and Akahori agreed that Japan and the Global Fund would continue further cooperation for the realization of UHC and the strengthening of health systems to prepare for future pandemic.[23]

In recent years, the total number of those who have suffered from HIV/AIDS infection in Japan has been on the increase since the 1980s, and amounted to 32,480 by the end of 2020, but early detection enables HIV/AIDS patients to be treated by medication.[24] On the other hand, some 260,000 people in Ukraine have suffered from HIV/AIDS, and medical service in the country has been disrupted due to Russia's invasion

---

[20] Ministry of Foreign Affairs of Japan. February 24, 2022. "Courtesy Call on Vice-Foreign Minister Takako Suzuki by Mr. Osamu Kunii as a Management Executive Committee Member of the Global Fund". https://www.mofa.go.jp/mofaj/ic/ghp/page1_001102.html.

[21] Ibid.

[22] Kunii, Osamu. 2019. *Sekai Saikyo Soshiki no Tsukurikata: Kansensho to Tatakau Global Fund no Chosen (How to Create the World's Strongest Organization: Challenge by the Global Fund to Fight Infectious Diseases).* Tokyo: Chikuma Shobo.

[23] Ministry of Foreign Affairs of Japan. April 9, 2022. "Meeting between Akahori Takeshi, Ambassador, Director-General for Global Issues of the Foreign Ministry and Mr. Peter Sands, Executive Director of the Global Fund". https://www.mofa.go.jp/mofaj/press/release/press1_000824.html.

[24] AIDS Prevention Information Network. 2020. "Annual Report on AIDS 2020". https://api-net.jfap.or.jp/status/japan/data/2020/nenpo/bunseki.pdf See also, National Institute of Infectious Diseases. 2018. "Acquired Immunodeficiency Syndrome, AIDS". https://www.niid.go.jp/niid/ja/kansennohanashi/400-aids-intro.html.

since February 24, 2022.[25] The Global Fund has been working together with the WHO and the United Nations Children's Fund (UNICEF) to address this issue in the war-affected country.

Nowadays, people in Japan tend to consider that tuberculosis is a disease of the past, but the number of those who are infected by tuberculosis has increased in Japan. In 2017, the Japanese government alerted that as many as 18,000 people were infected by tuberculosis every year in Japan, and some 1900 of them passed away owing to the disease each year.[26] According to the Ministry of Health, Labour and Welfare, 12,739 people in Japan were registered as patients of tuberculosis in 2020.[27] In Ukraine, approximately 30,000 people are infected by tuberculosis annually, and Anthony Fauci as Director of the National Institute of Allergy and Infectious Diseases in the United States warned that the Russian invasion of Ukraine would cause a serious tuberculosis problem as well as a "terrible public health tragedy".[28] Likewise, medical experts around the world have been concerned about "public health catastrophe" especially treatment for HIV/AIDS and tuberculosis in Ukraine.

According to the Cabinet Office, malaria was eradicated in Japan, and the final case of domestic infection of malaria was reported in Shiga Prefecture in 1959.[29] But, of late, Japanese people are being infected by the disease outside of the country. For Japanese people, malaria is still a travel-related infectious disease, but lethal nature of the disease cannot be underestimated. It was reported that 61 people in Japan were diagnosed with malaria in 2017, and 2 of them died. In 2019, 57 people in Japan

---

[25] UNAIDS. 2022. "Humanitarian Crisis: War in Ukraine". https://www.unaids.org/en.

[26] Government of Japan. 2017. "Be Alert for Old and New Disease, Tuberculosis!". https://www.gov-online.go.jp/useful/article/201509/3.html.

[27] Ministry of Health, Labour and Welfare of Japan. 2020. "Annual Report on the Registered Number of Tuberculosis Infection". https://www.mhlw.go.jp/stf/seisakunitsuite/bunya/0000175095_00004.html.

[28] Barbe, Harriet. March 5, 2022. "War in Ukraine Could Lead to 'Devastating' Tuberculosis Problem, Warns Anthony Fauci". *The Telegraph*. https://www.telegraph.co.uk/global-health/science-and-disease/war-ukraine-could-lead-devastating-tuberculosis-problem-warns/.

[29] Cabinet Office, Japan. March 26, 2008. "On Malaria". https://www.cao.go.jp/noguchisho/award/maraliafact.html.

were infected by malaria.[30] According to the US Centers for Disease Control and Prevention (CDC) moreover, some neighboring countries, such as China and South Korea, are categorized as malaria-endemic countries.[31] In this sense, the spread of malaria into Japan should not be overlooked in the progress of global warming as well as the globalization of tropical diseases. According to World Malaria Report 2021 publish by the WHO, 14 million more malaria cases and 47,000 more deaths in 2020 in comparison with 2019 were reported, indicating the negative impact of the coronavirus pandemic.[32] It indicates that Japan should continue to make further financial and diplomatic contributions to the Global Fund in the coronavirus pandemic period.

## Conclusion

Importantly, the rise in cases of the three major infectious diseases was influenced by the COVID-19 pandemic as discussed in this chapter. Moreover, HIV/AIDS and tuberculosis patients in Ukraine need continuous medical treatment in the middle of the Russia-Ukraine War that has disrupted ordinary medical services in the country. Hence, the international community, especially the Group of Seven (G7) member-states, is expected to take more proactive measures against the spread of the three major infectious diseases. On May 8, 2022, G7 leaders' online conference was held alongside Ukraine. In the "G7 Leaders Statement", it was confirmed that Russia's "illegal military aggression against Ukraine" has resulted in "terrible humanitarian catastrophe".[33] Without a doubt, the outbreak of the Russia-Ukraine War has damaged, aggravated, and devastated the public health system in Ukraine, and G7 countries including Japan are expected to make further contributions to the Global Fund.

[30] Osaka Institute of Public Health. April 19, 2021. "April 25 Is Malaria Day". http://www.iph.osaka.jp/li/070/20210419160926.html.

[31] Centers for Disease Control and Prevention (CDC). 2020. *Yellow Book 2020* (Chapter 4) https://wwwnc.cdc.gov/travel/yellowbook/2020/travel-related-infectious-diseases/malaria.

[32] World Health Organization (WHO). 2021. *World Malaria Report 2021.* https://www.who.int/teams/global-malaria-programme/reports/world-malaria-report-2021.

[33] Group of Seven (G7). May 8, 2022. "G7 Leaders' Statement". https://www.mofa.go.jp/mofaj/files/100341354.pdf.

TICAD 8 was an indispensable opportunity for the Japanese government to pledge its financial contribution to the Global Fund. In an official side event of TICAD 8 held on August 26, 2022, the Stop TB Partnership organized a meeting and published a report: "Securing the Finances to Save Lives in Africa from Tuberculosis". It is difficult to measure accurate impact of the advocacy by this official side event, but Lucica Ditiu as Executive Director of the Stop TB Partnership in cooperation with the World Bank Group discussed the necessity of funding opportunities and innovative financing with Japanese officials of the Ministry of Health, Labour and Welfare, Japan.[34]

In his opening speech of TICAD 8 held in Tunisia on August 27, 2022, Prime Minister Kishida stated that Japan would contribute up to 1.08 billion dollars to the Global Fund for the next three years in order to support the measures against the three major infectious diseases.[35] It is important to note that Kishida's decision on the pledge of the Global Fund at TICAD 8 was also encouraged by a multiparty parliamentary group, the Friends of the Global Fund, Japan Diet Task Force, requesting the Kishida government to pledge 1.1 billion dollars.[36] As an originator of the Global Fund, the Japanese government has consistently supported the activities of the Global Fund to control and eradicate the three major infectious diseases in the world. The Global Fund's Executive Director Sands noted that "Japan has proven that focusing intensely on fighting an infectious disease delivers much more than the benefit of halting that particular threat".[37] Having said that, Japan is still the fifth largest public donor to the Global Fund, following the United States,

[34] Stop TB Partnership. 2022. "Securing the Finances to Save Lives in Africa from Tuberculosis". https://www.stoptb.org/event/ticad-8-official-side-event.

[35] Ministry of Foreign Affairs of Japan. August 27, 2022. "Eighth Tokyo International Conference on African Development (TICAD 8) (Day 1: Opening Session and Plenary 1)". https://www.mofa.go.jp/afr/af2/page1e_000469.html.

[36] Friends of the Global Fund, Japan. August 3, 2022. "Ahead of the 7th Replenishment, Diet Task Force Members Submit a Letter to the Japanese Government Asking for a Strong Global Fund Pledge". https://fgfj.jcie.or.jp/en/news/diet-task-force-letter-2022/.

[37] Sands, Peter. July 14, 2023. "Japan's Fight Against TB Can Be a Roadmap for Pandemic Preparedness". The Global Fund. https://www.theglobalfund.org/en/opinion/2023/2023-07-14-japans-fight-against-tb-can-be-a-roadmap-for-pandemic-preparedness/.

France, the United Kingdon, and Germany.[38] Therefore, Japan as the fourth largest economy in the world is expected to make further financial and diplomatic contributions to the Global Fund toward TICAD 9 to be held in Yokohama in 2025.

[38] Kunii, Osamu. 2019. *Sekai Saikyo Soshiki no Tsukurikata: Kansensho to Tatakau Global Fund no Chosen (How to Create the World's Strongest Organization: Challenge by the Global Fund to Fight Infectious Diseases)*. Tokyo: Chikuma Shobo, p. 136.

# CHAPTER 4

# Japan and the GPEI: Toward a Polio-Free World

**Abstract** In the middle of the coronavirus pandemic, other infectious diseases, including poliovirus, are apt to be forgotten, but the significance of routine vaccination against preventable infectious diseases should not be underestimated. Poliovirus is an infectious disease that seriously affects human body. There used to be more than 125 countries which had suffered from wild poliovirus endemic in the 1980s. As a result of endeavors by the Global Polio Eradication Initiative (GPEI) established in 1988, the number of wild poliovirus endemic countries has been reduced to only two countries: Afghanistan and Pakistan. This chapter sheds light on the importance of Japan's contributions to poliovirus eradication by contextualizing Japan's experience in eradicating its own wild poliovirus, and Japan's financial contributions toward the GPEI in pursuit of a "polio-free" world.

**Keywords** Afghanistan · Global Polio Eradication Initiative (GPEI) · Japan · Pakistan · Polio (poliovirus)

D. Akimoto, *Japan and Global Health*, https://doi.org/10.1007/978-981-97-0972-4_4

## INTRODUCTION

In the middle of the COVID-19 pandemic, other infectious diseases, including poliovirus, are apt to be forgotten, but the significance of routine vaccination against preventable infectious diseases should not be underestimated even in the pandemic period. Poliomyelitis (polio or poliovirus) is an infectious disease that seriously affects human body. The virus invades the nervous system and may cause eternal paralysis of arms and legs to human beings, especially children under five years old.[1] In addition to the paralysis, polio-disabled people occasionally suffer from "discrimination as structural violence".[2] Human beings have suffered from polio since ancient times as illustrated in Pharaonic inscriptions in Egypt,[3] yet have attempted to control and eradicate the disease.

It is publicly known that polio is a "preventable" disease, but it is not necessarily widely recognized that polio is an "incurable" disease for human beings at this stage. According to the Japanese Ministry of Health, Labour and Welfare, children (basically from two-month-old to eighteen-month-old infants) in Japan are supposed to be vaccinated four times free of charge due to financial support by the government.[4] Most Japanese people have taken the routine poliovirus vaccination for granted, but the Japanese people suffered from outbreaks of polio in the past. Japan's response to the polio endemic in its country and the world has profound implications for the current coronavirus pandemic and its vaccine diplomacy.[5]

There used to be more than 125 countries which had suffered from wild poliovirus endemic in the 1980s. As a result of endeavors by the Global Polio Eradication Initiative (GPEI) established in 1988, the

[1] World Health Organization (WHO). 2022. "Poliomyelitis (Polio)". https://www.who.int/health-topics/poliomyelitis#tab=tab_1.

[2] Szántó, Diana. 2020. *Politicising Polio: Disability, Civil Society and Civic Agency in Sierra Leone*. Singapore: Palgrave Macmillan, pp. 153–183.

[3] United Nations Children's Fund (UNICEF). 2022. "Polio in Egypt". https://www.unicef.org/egypt/polio-egypt.

[4] Ministry of Health, Labour and Welfare of Japan. January 29, 2018. "Basic Information on Polio and Polio Vaccines". https://www.mhlw.go.jp/bunya/kenkou/polio/qa.html.

[5] Japan Times. February 17, 2022. "Japan Stepping up COVID Vaccine Diplomacy, without Strings Attached". https://www.japantimes.co.jp/news/2022/02/17/national/japan-covid19-vaccine-diplomacy/.

number of wild poliovirus endemic countries has been reduced to only two countries: Afghanistan and Pakistan. In other words, if the two countries in South Asia succeed in eradicating their wild poliovirus, wild poliovirus can be eradicated in the world. This chapter sheds light on the importance of Japan's contributions to poliovirus eradication by contextualizing Japan's experience in eradicating its own wild poliovirus, and Japan's financial contributions to global polio eradication toward the GPEI in pursuit of a "polio-free" world.[6]

## POLIO OUTBREAKS, VACCINE IMPORTS, AND ROUTINE VACCINATION IN JAPAN

Historically, occasional polio outbreaks in Japan became discernible after the termination of its isolationist foreign policy, namely the national seclusion policy. The cycle of the outbreaks of polio occurred in the 1910s, the 1920s, and the 1930s. In postwar Japan, a serious spread of polio occurred in Aomori in 1948.[7] The annual occurrence of polio cases between 1948 and 1959 was approximately 2000–3000 on average.[8] In 1960, another outbreak of polio occurred in Hokkaido, and the number of polio cases mounted to 5606, marking the worst record in Japan.[9] Outraged mothers, who were concerned about the health condition of their children, protested on the streets and besieged the Health and Welfare Ministry which was reluctant to import poliovirus vaccines, especially due to the lack of sufficient clinical evidence of possible side-effects.[10]

---

[6] This chapter is based on my earlier research on Japan's contribution to polio eradication. See, Akimoto, Daisuke. April 21, 2022. "Japan's Vaccine Diplomacy toward a 'Polio-Free' World". *ISDP Voices*. https://isdp.eu/japans-vaccine-diplomacy-toward-a-polio-free-world/.

[7] Katow, Shigetaka. 2010. "Polio". *Modern Media*. Vol. 56, No. 3, pp. 61–68. https://www.eiken.co.jp/uploads/modern_media/literature/MM1003_03.pdf.

[8] Takatsu, T., I. Tagaya, and M. Hirayama. 1973. "Poliomyelitis in Japan during the Period 1962–68 after the Introduction of Mass Vaccination with Sabin Vaccine". *Bulletin of World Health Organization*. Vol. 49, No. 2, pp. 129–137.

[9] Ibid.

[10] Yegorov, Oleg. January 21, 2021. "How the USSR Helped Japan Defeat a Deadly Virus". *Russia Beyond*. https://www.rbth.com/science-and-tech/333327-ussr-japan-polio-vaccine.

In June 1961, the Japanese government eventually decided to import oral poliovirus vaccine (OPV) mostly from the Soviet Union and partly from Canada, and mass vaccination was implemented in Japan despite the existence of concerns about side-effects.[11] Notably, Health and Welfare Minister Yoshimi Furui stated that he would take all responsibilities for the decision on the emergency import and mass vaccination in Japan. It is estimated that 13 million doses from the Soviet Union saved over 20 million Japanese children.[12] This was an unusual case of international cooperation between Tokyo and Moscow in the Cold War, but it was a result of the normalization of the bilateral diplomatic ties based on the Joint Declaration between Japan and the Soviet Union in 1956. During the 1960s, the number of polio patients drastically decreased owing to the mass vaccination.[13] As a result of the poliovirus control based on OPV, wild-type polio cases have never been reported since 1981 in Japan.[14]

Although routine vaccination of OPV was implemented and the elimination of wild poliovirus was achieved in Japan, polio cases among OPV recipients as vaccine-associated paralytic poliomyelitis (VAPP) continued to be reported every year, with the most in 2011.[15] According to a survey in Kanagawa, most parents replied that they thought OPV was not safe enough and desired their children to take inactivated poliovirus vaccine (IPV). The Japan Pediatric Society advised that children should take OPV until domestically produced IPV could be available. On the contrary, the World Health Organization (WHO) recommended that OPV should be

[11] Iskra Industry. 2001–2015. "History". http://www.iskra.co.jp/tabid/268/Default.aspx.

[12] Yegorov, Oleg. January 21, 2021. "How the USSR Helped Japan Defeat a Deadly Virus". *Russia Beyond*. https://www.rbth.com/science-and-tech/333327-ussr-japan-polio-vaccine.

[13] Infectious Disease Surveillance Center. 2012. "Reported Cases of Poliomyelitis in Japan, 1947–1994". https://idsc.niid.go.jp/iasr/18/203/graph/f203-1.gif.

[14] Shimojo, Hiroto. 1984. "Poliomyelitis Control in Japan". *Reviews of Infectious Diseases*. Vol. 6, Supplement 2, pp. 427–430.

[15] Miyoshi, Masahiro, Shima Yoshizumi, Masaru Jinushi, Setsuko Ishida, Toyo Okui, Motohiko Okano, Masayo Shouji, Sanae Tanaka, Junichi Saigusa, Akihisa Mori, Hiroki Tanabe, Ryo Yamaguchi, Yorihiro Nishimura, and Hiroyuki Shimizu. 2010. "A Case of Paralytic Poliomyelitis Associated with Poliovirus Vaccine Strains in Hokkaido, Japan". *Japanese Journal of Infectious Diseases*. Vol. 63, No. 3, pp. 216–217. For an analysis of VAPP, see also Hosoda, Miwako, Hajime Inoue, Yasuo Miyazawa, Eiji Kusumi, and Kenji Shibuya. 2012. "Vaccine-Associated Paralytic Poliomyelitis in Japan". *Lancet*. Vol. 379, No. 9815, p. 520.

replaced with IPV in countries that had achieved the poliovirus elimination. Japan was one of the few industrialized countries that used OPV even after the elimination of poliovirus in the country, and the Japanese public patiently demanded that the government replace OPV with IPV for domestic routine vaccination.[16] In the Committee on Health, Labour and Welfare of the House of Representatives held on March 8, 2011, Noriko Furuya of Komeito ardently requested the Japanese government to introduce IPV routine vaccination with the official financial support.[17] As a result of the tenacious advocacy for IPV routine vaccination, the Japanese government finally stopped the use of OPV and introduced IPV as of September 2012.

## JAPAN'S CONTRIBUTION TO THE GLOBAL POLIO ERADICATION INITIATIVE (GPEI)

In the meanwhile, Rotary International began its fight against polio by initiating a multi-year project to immunize six million children in the Philippines in 1979, and launched the first and largest internationally coordinated poliovirus eradication project, namely "PolioPlus" with an initial fundraising target of 120 million dollars in 1985.[18] In 1988, the World Health Assembly of the WHO adopted a resolution to launch the GPEI as a public–private partnership,[19] with international support by the WHO, Rotary International, the US Centers for Disease Control and Prevention (CDC), and the United Nations Children's Fund (UNICEF). The Bill & Melinda Gates Foundation (Gates Foundation) and Gavi, the Vaccine Alliance, later join the GPEI. Notably, the Japanese government

[16] Nakano, Takashi. 2011. "Japanese Vaccinations and Practices, with Particular Attention to Polio and Pertussis". *Travel Medicine and Infectious Disease*. Vol. 9, No. 4, pp. 169–175.

[17] National Diet Library. March 8, 2011. "Proceedings of the 177th Diet Session. The Committee on Health, Labour and Welfare, the House of Representatives". https://kokkai.ndl.go.jp/#/detail?minId=117704260X00320110308&spkNum=86&current=9.

[18] Rotary International. 2022. "Rotary and the Fight Against Polio". https://www.endpolio.org/rotary-and-the-fight-against-polio.

[19] World Health Organization (WHO). 2022. "Poliomyelitis (Polio)". https://www.who.int/health-topics/poliomyelitis#tab=tab_1.

has consistently made financial contributions toward the GPEI since its inception.[20]

Being encouraged by the global polio eradication movement, a non-partisan parliamentary association, the Diet Task Force on Global Polio Eradication, was established in Japan in May 2011. In August of the year, the Japanese government decided to initiate a poliovirus vaccination project as part of its official development assistance (ODA) to Pakistan by financing some five billion yen in cooperation with the Gates Foundation.[21] The polio eradication project was implemented by a loan conversion method, and the Gates Foundation agreed to repay the entire debt for Japan's ODA loan in place of the Pakistani government.[22] In September 2014, the Japan International Cooperation Agency (JICA) and the Gates Foundation agreed on another loan conversion contract to finance some eight billion yen for polio eradication in Nigeria.[23] Moreover, several projects by the JICA contributed to eradicating poliovirus in China through a bilateral collaboration as well as international cooperation.[24]

The epoch-making loan conversion method can be regarded as an integral part of Japan's global health policy,[25] and it is observed that

[20] Global Polio Eradication Initiative (GPEI). 2021. "Contributions and Pledges to the Global Polio Eradication Initiative, 1985–2020". https://polioeradication.org/wp-content/uploads/2021/07/GPEI_FIN_Historical-Contributions_Journals-Charts_asat_2 020-12-31.pdf.

[21] Ministry of Foreign Affairs of Japan. 2011. "Japan's Official Development Assistance White Paper 2011". https://www.mofa.go.jp/policy/oda/white/2011/html/keyword/keyword02.html.

[22] Japan Institute for Global Health (JIGH). 2011–2014. "Polio". http://jigh.org/en/activity/project/polio.html.

[23] Japan International Cooperation Agency (JICA). 2014. "JICA Signs Innovative Financing Agreement with Gates Foundation for Polio Eradication in Nigeria". https://www.jica.go.jp/usa/english/office/others/newsletter/2014/1409_10_02.html.

[24] Okada, Minoru. 2014. *Bokura no Mura kara Polio ga Kieta: Chugoku Santosho-hatsu "Kagakuteki Genjitsushugi" no Kokusai Kyoryoku (Poliovirus Disappeared from Our Village: International Cooperation of "Scientific Realism" in Shandong Province of China)*. Tokyo: Saiki Communications.

[25] Sugiyama, Haruko, Ayaka Yamaguchi, and Hiromi Murakami. 2013. *Japan's Global Health Policy: Developing a Comprehensive Approach in a Period of Economic Stress*. Edited by Katherine E. Bliss. New York: Rowman & Littlefield Publishers.

the polio immunization program in Nigeria contributed to polio eradication in Africa.[26] In July 2015, the Diet Task Force on Global Polio Eradication submitted a "resolution to support polio eradication for children in the world" to Vice-Foreign Minister Yasuhide Nakayama.[27] Since then, Tokyo has made financial contributions including grant aid assistance to polio vaccination programs led by the UNICEF in Afghanistan,[28] Pakistan,[29] Nigeria, and the Lake Chad region.[30] In October 2015, a delegation of the Diet Task Force on Global Polio Eradication visited Pakistan in order to inspect the site of poliovirus vaccination and have talks with the health minister and other politicians in the country regarding the issue of polio eradication.[31]

During the administration of former Prime Minister Shinzo Abe, the Japanese government made significant contributions to the GPEI, and Rotary International granted the Polio Eradication Champion Award to Abe in 2015. Abe also played a central role in reconfirming Japan's commitment to polio eradication at the pledge event of the Rotary

[26] Craig, Allen S., Rustam Haydarov, Helena O'Malley, Michael Galway, Halima Dao, Ngashi Ngongo, Marie Therese Baranyikwa, Savita Naqvi, Nima S. Abid, Carol Pandak, and Amy Edwards. 2017 "The Public Health Legacy of Polio Eradication in Africa". *Journal of Infectious Diseases*. Vol. 216, No. 1, pp. 343–350.

[27] Japan Institute for Global Health (JIGH). August 4, 2015. "A Resolution to Support Polio Eradication for Children in the World" Submitted to Vice-Foreign Minister Yasuhide Nakayama". http://jigh.org/news/jigh/2390.

[28] United Nations Children's Fund (UNICEF). November 27, 2017. "Japan Donates 17.7 Million USD to Provide Life-saving Vaccines for Children in Afghanistan". https://www.unicef.org/tokyo/news/2017/japan-donates-17.7-million-usd-to-provide-life-saving-vaccines-for-children-in-afghanistan.

[29] United Nations Children's Fund (UNICEF). December 13, 2021. "Japan Announces New US$ 4.35 Million Grant to Support Polio Programme in Pakistan". https://www.unicef.org/tokyo/news/2021/japan-announces-new-us-435-million-grant-support-polio-programme-pakistan.

[30] United Nations Children's Fund (UNICEF). February 16, 2017. "Japan Gives $33.3 Million in Emergency Funding to Nigeria and Lake Chad Region". https://www.unicef.org/tokyo/news/2017/japan-gives-33.3-million-in-emergency-funding-to-protect-children-from-polio-in-nigeria-and-lake-chad-region.

[31] National Diet Library. March 21, 2017. "Proceedings of the 193rd Diet Session. Special Committee on Official Development Assistance, etc., the House of Councillors". https://kokkai.ndl.go.jp/#/detail?minId=119314580X00220170321&spkNum=26&current=2.

Convention held in Atlanta in 2017.[32] During the Special Committee on Official Development Assistance, etc. held in the House of Councillors on March 21, 2017, Kenzo Fujisue from the Democratic Party of Japan as secretariat of the Diet Task Force on Global Polio Eradication pointed out the significance of Japan's financial contribution toward polio eradication. In response, Koichi Aiboshi as a government official explained that Japan had made contributions to the GPEI as well as the loan conversion method in collaboration with the Gates Foundation.[33]

## POLIOVIRUS RECURRENCE AND THE SIGNIFICANCE OF JAPAN'S VACCINE DIPLOMACY

Through the endeavor of the polio vaccination program within the framework of the GPEI, it was confirmed in 2019 that there had been no polio cases in Nigeria for three years, and the WHO declared in August 2020 that wild poliovirus had been eradicated in Africa.[34] After the declaration of the polio-free African continent, Afghanistan and Pakistan became the last two remaining countries as the final poliovirus bastions, where wild poliovirus still exists.[35] On November 19, 2020, Kenzo Fujisue reported on his blog that the Diet Task Force on Global Polio Eradication took place for the first time in two years, highlighting the polio-free declaration in Africa of the year.[36] On February 17, 2022 however, the WHO declared an outbreak of a polio case of a three-year-old girl as the first

[32] Global Polio Eradication Initiative (GPEI). July 13, 2022. "In Remembrance of the Former Prime Minister of Japan, Hon. Shinzo Abe". https://polioeradication.org/news-post/in-remembrance-of-the-former-prime-minister-of-japan-hon-shinzo-abe/.

[33] National Diet Library. March 21, 2017. "Proceedings of the 193rd Diet Session. Special Committee on Official Development Assistance, etc., the House of Councillors". https://kokkai.ndl.go.jp/#/detail?minId=119314580X00220170321&spkNum=27&current=1.

[34] UN News Center. 2022. "Polio Is No Longer Endemic in Nigeria: UN Health Strategy". https://www.un.org/africarenewal/news/polio-no-longer-endemic-nigeria---un-health-agency.

[35] World Health Organization (WHO). January 4, 2019. "Pakistan and Afghanistan: The Final Wild Poliovirus Bastion". https://www.who.int/news-room/feature-stories/detail/pakistan-and-afghanistan-the-final-wild-poliovirus-bastion.

[36] Kenzo Fujisue Official Blog. November 19, 2020. "The Diet Task Force on Global Polio Eradication Was Held". https://ameblo.jp/fujisue-kenzo/entry-12644410496.html.

case in five years in the "polio-free" African continent.[37] The strain found in the Malawian girl reportedly stemmed from Pakistan, and this incident indicates the difficulty in preventing the cross-border spread of poliovirus. The case in Malawi also suggests that any countries including Japan could have a new polio case owing to globalization.

In the middle of the COVID-19 pandemic, the number of children who took routine vaccinations decreased in Japan and the world.[38] In fact, the WHO and the CDC warned that the largest decrease was in the number of children vaccinated for measles during the pandemic period.[39] In the case of polio vaccination, it is necessary for children to take vaccine shots several times for sufficient immunization. As mentioned earlier, children in Japan are allowed to take IPV four times in total free of charge due to the official financial support, but children in some European countries including the United Kingdom, Germany, and France, are supposed to take five doses of polio vaccines as reported by Sanofi Pasteur.[40]

Since possibilities of a re-outbreak of poliovirus in Japan, stemming from unvaccinated people overseas, cannot be ruled out, an additional fifth dose of IPV may be necessary for children in Japan as deliberated in the Ministry of Health, Labour and Welfare and encouraged by some requests from the private sector.[41] In fact, the UK Health Security Agency announced on June 22, 2022, that poliovirus had been detected in sewage

[37] World Health Organization (WHO). February 17, 2022. "Malawi Declares Polio Outbreak". https://www.afro.who.int/news/malawi-declares-polio-outbreak.

[38] Kumai, Hiromi. June 26, 2020. "Routine Vaccination Rate of Three-Year-Old Children Decreased". *Asahi Shimbun.* https://www.asahi.com/articles/ASN6T5JMFN6LULB J01X.html.

[39] World Health Organization (WHO). December 10, 2021. "Global Progress against Measles Threatened amidst COVID-19 Pandemic". https://www.who.int/news/item/ 10-11-2021-global-progress-against-measles-threatened-amidst-covid-19-pandemic.

[40] Sanofi Pasteur. 2019. "Imovax Polio". https://e-mr.sanofi.co.jp/-/media/EMS/ Conditions/eMR/leaflet/pdf/IPV_19_08_0169.pdf. See also, Ministry of Health, Labour and Welfare of Japan. 2016. "IPV Vaccination Schedule in Other Countries". https://www.mhlw.go.jp/file/05-Shingikai-10601000-Daijinkanboukouseikagakuka-Kou seikagakuka/0000145361.pdf.

[41] Ministry of Health, Labour and Welfare of Japan. 2016. "Fifth Dose of IPV". https://www.mhlw.go.jp/file/05-Shingikai-10601000-Daijinkanboukouseikag akuka-Kouseikagakuka/0000145358.pdf.

from North and East London,[42] and the agency declared a rare "national incidence" for the first time in nearly 40 years.[43] Similarly, it was reported on *CNN* on July 22, 2022, an unvaccinated young adult had been diagnosed with poliovirus for the first time in the United States in nearly a decade.[44] Poliovirus detection in metropolitan cities, such as London and New York, indicates that poliovirus detection in other major cities including Tokyo cannot be ruled out. In 1981, a poliovirus was detected from wastes of a jetliner at Narita Airport,[45] and therefore, it is still possible that poliovirus can be transported by international airlines from overseas countries to Japan.

By implementing proper routine polio vaccination with IPV, Japan can save the lives of children in the country. At the event of the Eighth Tokyo International Conference on African Development (TICAD 8) held in Tunisia on August, 27–28 2022,[46] the Kishida administration discussed how to make further diplomatic and financial contributions to facilitating the achievement of a "polio-free world" in the midst of the COVID-19 pandemic.[47] In the TICAD 8, it was confirmed that Japan had contributed some 117 billion yen to Gavi and 18.7 billion yen to the Coalition for Epidemic Preparedness Innovations (CEPI) so that

---

[42] The UK Government. June 22, 2022. "Poliovirus Detected in Sewage from North and East London". https://www.gov.uk/government/news/poliovirus-detected-in-sewage-from-north-and-east-london.

[43] Harris, Rob. June 23, 2022. "Poliovirus Detected in London Sewage, National Incident Declared". *Sydney Morning Herald*. https://www.smh.com.au/world/europe/polio-virus-detected-in-london-sewage-national-incident-declared-20220623-p5avw2.html.

[44] Goodman, Brenda. July 22, 2022. "New York Adult Diagnosed with Polio, First US Case in Nearly a Decade". *CNN*. https://edition.cnn.com/2022/07/21/health/new-york-polio/index.html.

[45] Yoneyama, Tetsuo, Takashi Fujiwara, Yoko Yokota, Yoshimi Takemika, and Akio Hagiwara. 1995. "Characterization of a Wild Poliovirus Type 3 Isolated in Japan in 1993". *Japanese Journal of Medical Science and Biology*. Vol. 48, No. 1, pp. 61–70.

[46] Ministry of Foreign Affairs of Japan. February 8, 2022. "The Eighth Tokyo International Conference on African Development (TICAD 8) (Tunisia)". https://www.mofa.go.jp/afr/af2/page24e_000325.html.

[47] TICAD Monitor.org. 2022. "TICAD 8 Tunis Plan of Actions: Actions for Implementation of TICAD 8 Tunis Plan of Actions". https://ticad-monitor.org/wp-content/uploads/ENG-TICAD-8-Tunis-Plan-of-Actions.pdf.

about 800,000 children could be vaccinated as measures against infectious diseases, including poliovirus.[48]

Meanwhile, a meeting of the Diet Task Force on Global Polio Eradication was held on October 13, 2022. Despite the pandemic period, a number of Diet members attended the nonpartisan meeting, although there was no secretariat of the task force since Kenzo Fujisue lost his seat in the Diet as a result of the Upper House election held in July 2022. As a former secretariat of the task force, Kenzo Fujisue attended the meeting and reported on his official blog on the 2022–2026 GPEI Strategy that targets vaccination for 370 million children.[49] Rio Tomonoh of the LDP as a mother of children with background of a nurse and lawyer attended the meeting of the task force for the first time.[50] In this sense, it is important for the Diet Task Force on Global Polio Eradication to increase the number of members of the task force to strengthen its organizational and political influence. As Fujisue discussed in the Diet, Japan's ODA was used for constructing a factory to create poliovirus vaccines in Indonesia,[51] and therefore, Japan's financial contributions to the GPEI as well as ODA to other countries are of significance in the process of polio eradication in the world.

In this context, the Japanese government pledged 11 million dollars to the GPEI's 2022–2026 Strategy at the event of the World Health Summit (WHS) held in Berlin, Germany on October 18, 2023.[52] Japan's financial contribution to the GPEI's strategy announced at the WHS was meaningful, yet other donor countries and organizations also pledged their financial contributions: Australia pledged 43.55 million Australian

---

[48] Ibid.

[49] Kenzo Fujisue Official Blog. October 13, 2022. "Distributing Vaccines to the Children in the World: The Diet Task Force on Global Polio Eradication Was Held". https://ameblo.jp/fujisue-kenzo/entry-12769308034.html.

[50] Rio Tomonoh Official Site. October 15, 2022. "Daily Activity Report". https://tomonoh.net/activity-report135/.

[51] National Diet Library. March 21, 2017. "Proceedings of the 193rd Diet Session. Special Committee on Official Development Assistance, etc., the House of Councillors". https://kokkai.ndl.go.jp/#/detail?minId=119314580X00220170321&spkNum=26&current=2.

[52] World Health Organization (WHO). October 18, 2022. "Global Leaders Commit US$ 2.6 Billion at World Health Summit to End Polio". https://www.who.int/news/item/18-10-2022-global-leaders-commit-usd-2.6-billion-at-world-health-summit-to-end-polio.

dollars, France pledged 50 million euro, Germany pledged 72 million euro, Republic of Korea pledged 4.5 billion won, Luxembourg pledged 1.7 million euro, Malta pledged 30,000 euro, Monaco pledged 450,000 euro, Spain pledged 100,000 euro, Turkey pledged 20,000 dollars, United States pledged 114 million dollars, the Gates Foundation pledged 1.2 billion dollars, Bloomberg Philanthropies pledged 50 million dollars, Islamic Food and Nutrition Council of America pledged 1.8 million dollars, Latter-day Saint Charities pledged 400,000 dollars, Rotary International pledged 150 million dollars, and UNICEF pledged 5 million dollars.[53] Thanks to the polio immunization programs by the Rotary International and the GPEI, the number of polio cases has been drastically reduced since the 1980s as shown in Fig. 4.1.[54] Nevertheless, the number of polio cases mostly occurred in countries of Southeast Asia, especially Afghanistan and Pakistan.

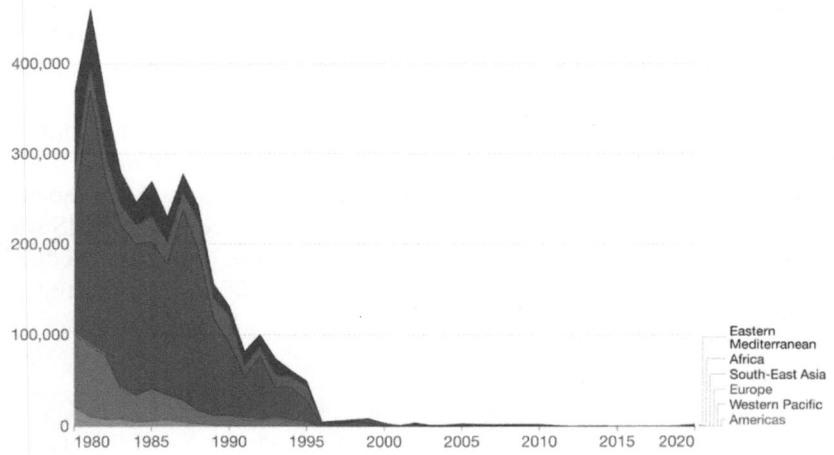

**Fig. 4.1** Paralytic polio: estimated cases by World Region 1980–2020 (*Note* Source by Saloni Dattani, Fiona Spooner, Sophie Ochmann, and Max Roser 2022)

[53] Ibid.

[54] Dattani, Saloni, Fiona Spooner, Sophie Ochmann, and Max Roser. 2022. "Polio". *Our World in Data* (First published in November 2017 and last updated in April 2022). https://ourworldindata.org/polio.

## Japan's Contributions to Polio Vaccination in Afghanistan and Pakistan

In conjunction with the GPEI, the Japanese government has made financial contributions to eradicating wild poliovirus in Afghanistan and Pakistan. Japan's bilateral financial contributions to eradicating wild poliovirus in the South Asian countries have been made by the Ministry of Foreign Affairs through the UNICEF. Poliovirus immunization activities in Afghanistan have been in progress despite operational difficulties, such as "management and accountability problems in the field, inaccessible populations, and inadequate social mobilization".[55]

Why does Japan need to make financial contributions to polio eradication in Afghanistan and Pakistan? In terms of so-called "human development index" (HDI) based on a "summary measure of average achievement in key dimensions of human development: a long and healthy life, being knowledgeable and having a decent standard of living" annually announced by the United Nations Development Programme (UNDP),[56] the HDI of Afghanistan and Pakistan is considerably low in the world as shown in Table 4.1.[57] Clearly, the HDI ranking of both countries is categorized as "low human development" out of 191 countries. In cooperation with the international community, the Japanese government is responsible for financially supporting the two polio endemic countries in South Asia for this reason.

Indeed, Japan's financial contributions to polio eradication in Afghanistan and Pakistan have been consistent in the past. On December 10, 2011, it was announced that the Japanese government had provided 716 million yen with Afghanistan as a grant aid through the UNICEF

---

[55] Simpson, Diane M., Nahad Sadr-Azodi, Taufiq Mashal, Wrishmeen Sabawoon, Ajmal Pardis, Arshad Quddus, Carmen Garrigos, Sherine Guirguis, Syed Sohail Zahoor Zaidi, Shahzad Shaukat, Salmaan Sharif, Humayan Asghar, and Stephen C Hadler. 2014. "Polio Eradication Initiative in Afghanistan, 1997–2013". *Journal of Infectious Diseases*. Vol. 210, No. 1, pp. 162–172.

[56] United Nations Development Programme (UNDP). 2023. "Human Development Index (HDI)". https://hdr.undp.org/data-center/human-development-index#/indicies/HDI.

[57] United Nations Development Programme (UNDP). 2023. "HDI Dataset". https://hdr.undp.org/data-center/human-development-index#/indicies/HDI.

**Table 4.1** Comparison of the HDI of Afghanistan and Pakistan in 2021

|  | HDI rank | HDI (value) | Life expectancy at birth (years) | Expected years of schooling (years) | GNI per capita (dollars) |
|---|---|---|---|---|---|
| Afghanistan | 180 | 0.478 | 62.0 | 10.3 | 1824 |
| Pakistan | 161 | 0.544 | 66.1 | 8.7 | 4624 |

*Note* Statistical Data by the UNDP compiled by the author

for the purpose of wild poliovirus eradication.[58] On December 11, 2012, the UNICEF announced that the Japanese government had pledged to provide 1.06 billion yen (13 million dollars) for polio eradication and diseases prevention in Afghanistan.[59] On February 9, 2014, the government pledged 1.18 billion yen (12 million dollars) as a grant aid for polio eradication and diseases prevention in Afghanistan.[60] On January 21, 2015, the Ministry of Foreign Affairs of Japan announced that the government had pledged to provide 1.44 billion yen as a grant aid for the "project for infectious diseases for children" in Afghanistan through the UNICEF.[61]

On February 17, 2016, the Japanese government decided to make a financial contribution to polio eradication and diseases prevention in Afghanistan by providing 1.74 billion yen with the country through the UNICEF.[62] On December 13, 2016, it was announced that Japan had pledged 12.4 million dollars as a grant aid to Afghanistan for polio

[58] United Nations Children's Fund (UNICEF). December 10, 2011. "The Japanese Government Implemented 716 Million Yen Support for Polio Eradication in Afghanistan through the UNICEF". https://www.unicef.org/tokyo/news/2011/Dec-10.

[59] United Nations Children's Fund (UNICEF). December 11, 2012. "The Japanese Government Pledged 13 Million Dollars for Polio Eradication and Diseases Prevention in Afghanistan". https://www.unicef.org/tokyo/news/2012/Dec-11.

[60] United Nations Children's Fund (UNICEF). February 9, 2014. "The Japanese Government Decided on Support of 12 Million Dollars for Polio Eradication and Diseases Prevention through the UNICEF". https://www.unicef.org/tokyo/news/2014/Feb-9.

[61] Ministry of Foreign Affairs of Japan. January 21, 2015. "Exchange of Notes on Grant Aid to the 'Project for Infectious Diseases Prevention for Children' in Afghanistan through the UNICEF". https://www.mofa.go.jp/mofaj/press/release/press4_001678.html.

[62] United Nations Children's Fund (UNICEF). February 17, 2016. "The Japanese Government Decided on Support of 1.748 Billion Yen for Diseases Prevention of Children in Afghanistan through the UNICEF". https://www.unicef.org/tokyo/news/2016/Feb-17.

eradication and diseases prevention in the country.[63] On November 17, 2017, the government announced to donate 17.7 million dollars to provide life-saving vaccines for children to eradicate wild poliovirus and prevent infectious diseases in Afghanistan.[64] On December 3, 2018, Japan pledged to provide 9.1 million dollars as a grant aid to provide polio vaccines for children in Afghanistan through the UNICEF.[65]

On December 4, 2019, Japan donated 7 million dollars to support children and mother's health as well as polio eradication in Afghanistan.[66] On November 10, 2020, the Japanese government pledged to donate 940 million yen (approximately 9 million dollars) to support children and mother's health as well as polio eradication.[67] On May 19, 2022, the government announced to contribute 10.4 million dollars to the UNICEF in Afghanistan for proper immunization and polio eradication of the country.[68] On March 26, 2023, it was announced that

---

[63] United Nations Children's Fund (UNICEF). December 13, 2016. "Government of Japan Commits US$ 12.4 Million to Provide Life-saving Vaccines in Afghanistan". https://www.unicef.org/tokyo/news/2016/government-of-japan-commits-us-12.4-million-to-provide-life-saving-vaccines-and-prevent-the-spread-of-infectious-diseases-in-afghanistan.

[64] United Nations Children's Fund (UNICEF). November 17, 2017. "Japan Donates 17.7 Million USD to Provide Life-saving Vaccines for Children in Afghanistan". https://www.unicef.org/tokyo/news/2017/japan-donates-17.7-million-usd-to-provide-life-saving-vaccines-for-children-in-afghanistan.

[65] United Nations Children's Fund (UNICEF). December 3, 2018. "Japan Donates US$9.1 Million to Support Children and Mother's Health in Afghanistan". https://www.unicef.org/afghanistan/press-releases/japan-donates-us91-million-support-children-and-mothers-health-afghanistan.

[66] United Nations Children's Fund (UNICEF). December 4, 2019. "UNICEF Welcomes Japan's USD 7 Million Contribution to Support Children and Mother's Health in Afghan". https://www.unicef.org/tokyo/news/2019/unicef-welcomes-japan%E2%80%99s-usd-7-million-contribution-to-support-children-and-mother%E2%80%99s-health-in-afghan.

[67] United Nations Children's Fund (UNICEF). November 10, 2020. "Japan Provides Approximately 9 Million USD to Support Children and Mother's Health in Afghanistan". https://www.unicef.org/tokyo/news/2020/press-releases/japan-provides-approximately-9-million-usd-support-children-and-mothers-health.

[68] United Nations Children's Fund (UNICEF). May 19, 2022. "Japan Contributes US$ 10.4 Million to UNICEF Afghanistan for Administration of Essential Vaccines". https://www.unicef.org/tokyo/news/2022/japan-contributes-us-104-million-unicef-afghanistan-administration-essential.

Japan would contribute over 3 billion yen (21 million dollars) to vaccination program including polio vaccination, water as well as sanitation in Afghanistan.[69] Thus, although Japan's financial contribution to polio vaccination program in Afghanistan was temporarily disrupted in 2021, Japan has been continuously committed to the eradication of poliovirus in the countries through the UNICEF.

Likewise, Japan has consistently made financial contributions to polio eradication endeavors in Pakistan. On November 3, 2011, Japan pledged to provide 23 million yen commensurate with 11 million doses of OPV for immunization activities in the country.[70] On March 11, 2013, the Ministry of Foreign Affairs announced that Japan had decided to contribute 226 million yen to the "project for the control and eradication of poliomyelitis" in Pakistan.[71] On March 7, 2014, the Japanese government announced to donate 389 million yen to the project for the control and eradication of poliomyelitis in Pakistan.[72] On November 17 of the year, Japan decided to donate 562 million yen commensurate with 15 million doses of OPV and 1.3 million doses of IPV to polio immunization activities in Pakistan through the UNICEF.[73] On March 15, 2016, the government decided to contribute 360 million yen to polio vaccination campaign in Pakistan through the UNICEF.[74] On November 29 of the year, Japan agreed to donate additional 44 million yen commensurate with 3.9 million doses of IPV to the polio vaccination campaign in

[69] United Nations Children's Fund (UNICEF). March 26, 2023. "Government of Japan Contributes over US$21 Million for Vaccines and WASH in Afghanistan's Schools". https://www.unicef.org/tokyo/news/2023/government-japan-contributes-over-us-21-million-life-saving-vaccines-and-water-and-sanitation-in-afghanistans-schools.

[70] United Nations Children's Fund (UNICEF). November 3, 2011. "The Japanese Government Contributes 23 Million Yen to Pakistan through UNICEF". https://www.unicef.org/tokyo/news/2011/Nov-3.

[71] Ministry of Foreign Affairs of Japan. March 11, 2013. "Exchange of Notes Signing Ceremony for the Grant Aid Project for the Project for the Control and Eradication of Poliomyelitis". https://www.mofa.go.jp/mofaj/press/release/25/3/0311_06.html.

[72] Ministry of Foreign Affairs of Japan. March 7, 2014. "Exchange of Notes Signing Ceremony for the Grant Aid Project for the Project for the Control and Eradication of Poliomyelitis". https://www.mofa.go.jp/mofaj/press/release/press4_000698.html.

[73] United Nations Children's Fund (UNICEF). November 17, 2014. "The Japanese Government Implements 562 Million Yen Support for Polio Eradication in Pakistan". https://www.unicef.org/tokyo/news/2014/Nov-17.

[74] United Nations Children's Fund (UNICEF). March 15, 2016. "The Japanese Government Decided on 360 Million Yen Support for Polio Eradication in Pakistan". https://www.unicef.org/tokyo/news/2016/Mar-15.

Pakistan through the UNICEF.[75] It was noteworthy that Japan's donation was used for IPV in Pakistan, since IPV tends to be used after eradication of wild poliovirus by OPV immunization campaign.

On October 18, 2017, the Japanese government announced to donate 520 million yen commensurate with 28 million doses of OPV for polio immunization activities in Pakistan.[76] Japan pledged to donate 510 million yen commensurate with 25 million doses of OPV for polio vaccination campaign in Pakistan on November 19, 2018.[77] On December 11, 2019, Japan donated 485 million yen for polio immunization campaign in Pakistan.[78] On January 27, 2021, Japan pledged to donate 484 million yen (4.57 million dollars) for OPV procurement in Pakistan. Kuninori Matsuda, Japanese Ambassador to Pakistan, stated that "Japan remains committed to assisting the people of Pakistan together with UNICEF in their goal of eradicating polio" even in the middle of the coronavirus pandemic.[79] On December 13 of the year, Japan pledge to donate additional 495 million yen (4.35 million dollars) as a grant aid for polio immunization program in Pakistan.[80] On December 8, 2022, the

[75] United Nations Children's Fund (UNICEF). November 29, 2016. "The Japanese Government Decided on 4.4 Million Yen Contribution to IPV Procurement in Support of Polio Eradication in Pakistan". https://www.unicef.org/tokyo/news/2016/japan-renews-commitment-to-support-polio-eradication-in-pakistan-japanese.

[76] United Nations Children's Fund (UNICEF). October 18, 2017. "The Japanese Government Decided on 520 Million Yen Contribution to Polio Eradication in Pakistan". https://www.unicef.org/tokyo/news/2017/japan-provides-520-million-yen-to-assist-pakistans-efforts-for-polio-eradication-japanese.

[77] United Nations Children's Fund (UNICEF). November 19, 2018. "The Japanese Government Decided on 510 Million Yen Contribution to OPV Procurement in Support of Polio Eradication in Pakistan". https://www.unicef.org/tokyo/news/2018/japan-provides-510-million-yen-to-assist-pakistans-efforts-for-polio-eradication-new-us-4.6-million-japanese-grant-to-procure-oral-polio-vaccine-japanese.

[78] United Nations Children's Fund (UNICEF). December 11, 2019. "Japan Renews Support for Polio Eradication Programme in Pakistan". https://www.unicef.org/tokyo/news/2019/japan-renews-support-for-polio-eradication-programme-in-pakistan.

[79] United Nations Children's Fund (UNICEF). January 27, 2021. "Japan Renews Commitment to Support Polio Eradication Efforts in Pakistan". https://www.unicef.org/tokyo/news/2021/japan-renews-commitment-to-support-polio-eradication-efforts-in-pakistan.

[80] United Nations Children's Fund (UNICEF). December 13, 2021. "Japan Announces New US$ 4.35 Million Grant to Support Polio Programme in Pakistan". https://www.unicef.org/tokyo/news/2021/japan-announces-new-us-435-million-grant-support-polio-programme-pakistan.

Japanese government provided 536 million yen (3.87 million dollars) as a grant with the Pakistani government for polio eradication program in the country.[81] As exemplified in the cases of bilateral financial contributions to Afghanistan and Pakistan, Japan has made consistent contributions to the polio eradication activities in the world, especially the two polio endemic countries in South Asia.

As shown in Table 4.2 moreover, Japan's bilateral financial contribution to polio eradication activities in Afghanistan and Pakistan had been consistent for 11 years from 2013 to 2023 excluding temporary disruption. On average, Japan's donations to polio vaccination programs through the UNICEF to Afghanistan and Pakistan are respectively 1.18 billion yen and 0.44 billion yen.[82] Now that the Taliban regime admitted the effectiveness and necessity of polio immunization campaigns,[83] the international community, especially the GPEI, is expected to make more contributions to the polio eradication activities in the two polio endemic countries in South Asia, toward a polio-free world.

**Table 4.2** Japan's contribution to Polio Eradication in Afghanistan and Pakistan 2013–2023

|  | 2013 | 2014 | 2015 | 2016 | 2017 | 2018 | 2019 | 2020 | 2021 | 2022 | 2023 |
|---|---|---|---|---|---|---|---|---|---|---|---|
| Afghanistan | N/A | 1.18 | 1.44 | 3.01 | 0.97 | 1.00 | 0.75 | 0.94 | N/A | 1.20 | 2.5 |
| Pakistan | 0.22 | 0.95 | N/A | 0.76 | 0.52 | 0.51 | 0.48 | N/A | 0.97 | 0.53 | N/A |

*Note* Excluding emergency grants other than polio. Data by the UNICEF (unit = billion yen)

[81] United Nations Children's Fund (UNICEF). December 8, 2022. "Japan Provides US$ 3.87 Million New Grants for Polio Eradication Efforts in Pakistan". https://www.unicef.org/tokyo/news/2022/japan-provides-us-3.87-million-new-grants-polio-eradication-efforts-pakistan.

[82] The average contribution to Pakistan from 2013 to 2022 is 0.49 billion yen as of December 24, 2023.

[83] Aljazeera. March 14, 2023. "Taliban Launches Annual Polio Vaccination Drive in Afghanistan". https://www.aljazeera.com/news/2023/3/14/taliban-launches-annual-polio-vaccination-drive-in-afghanistan.

## CONCLUSION

As scrutinized in this chapter, Japan's global health policy toward the global polio eradication activities by the GPEI has been consistent. Japan's own experience of poliovirus during the postwar period while containing and eradicating wild polio virus in the country indicates that large-scale and continuous poliovirus immunization campaigns are effective and necessary for eradicating the disease in Afghanistan and Pakistan. As part of its indirect financial contributions to the GPEI, Japan has made financial contributions to the two polio endemic countries in South Asia. The Japanese government has regarded the bilateral contributions to the two countries through the UNICEF as significant, but Japan's direct financial contributions to the GPEI should be regarded as important as the bilateral financial assistance to Afghanistan and Pakistan.

Given the HDI of Afghanistan and Pakistan, the Japanese government, in cooperation with the international community as well as the GPEI, is responsible for making financial contributions to eradicating wild poliovirus in the two countries. Moreover, detection of poliovirus in major cities, such as London and New York, suggests that Tokyo is not an exception in the spread of poliovirus in this globalized society. Notably, as the WHO declared on May 4, 2023 that COVID-19 "no longer constitutes a public health emergency of international concern (PHEIC)",[84] polio is the world's only infectious disease designated as the PHEIC status.[85] In order to protect children and people in Japan and the world, the Japanese government, in conjunction with the international community, is expected to make further diplomatic and financial contributions to eradicating poliovirus in Afghanistan and Pakistan toward a polio-free world.

---

[84] World Health Organization (WHO). May 5, 2023. "Statement on the Fifteenth Meeting of the IHR (2005) Emergency Committee on the COVID-19 Pandemic". https://www.who.int/news/item/05-05-2023-statement-on-the-fifteenth-meeting-of-the-international-health-regulations-(2005)-emergency-committee-regarding-the-corona virus-disease-(covid-19)-pandemic.

[85] World Health Organization (WHO). September 7, 2023. "Polio: As of Today, the World's Only Public Health Emergency of International Concern". https://www.emro. who.int/polio-eradication/news/polio-as-of-today-the-worlds-only-public-health-emerge ncy-of-international-concern.html.

# CHAPTER 5

# Japan's TICAD Diplomacy for Global Health in Africa

**Abstract** The Japanese government has made diplomatic contributions to development and global health of the African continent by holding the Tokyo International Conference on African Development (TICAD). The initiation of the TICAD diplomacy was 1993 prior to the adoption of its human security policy as a diplomatic pillar. Why is Tokyo motivated to contribute to the development of the African continent? To understand Japan's approach and motivations for its Africa diplomacy, it is necessary to contextualize and examine the TICAD processes and keynote speeches given by successive Japanese prime ministers. This chapter clarifies the consistency of Japan's commitment to the TICAD conferences as well as Japan's strategic motivations to pursue its strategic foreign policy vision, namely Free and Open Indo-Pacific (FOIP) in recent years.

**Keywords** Abe · Africa · Free and Open Indo-pacific (FOIP) · Japan · Tokyo International Conference on African Development (TICAD)

© The Author(s), under exclusive license to Springer Nature
Singapore Pte Ltd. 2024
D. Akimoto, *Japan and Global Health*,
https://doi.org/10.1007/978-981-97-0972-4_5

## Introduction

The Japanese government has made diplomatic contributions to global health by holding international conferences on development of the African continent. The Tokyo International Conference on African Development (TICAD) has been held by the Japanese government in affiliation with the United Nations, the United Nations Development Program (UNDP), the African Union, and the World Bank since 1993. Since then, the Japanese governments have made continuous contributions to the development of Africa through the TICAD diplomacy. Why is Tokyo motivated to contribute to the development of the African continent? To understand Japan's approach and motivations, it is necessary to contextualize and examine the TICAD process and keynote speeches given by successive Japanese prime ministers.[1]

As for earlier research on Japan's TICAD diplomacy, Howard Lehman examined Japan's foreign aid policy to Africa through the TICAD initiative.[2] Bert Edström chronologically investigated Japan's policy toward the TICAD process in *Asia Paper* published by the Institute for Security and Development Policy (ISDP).[3] Pedro Amakasu Raposo, currently a professor at Kansai University, published a book, *Japan's Foreign Aid Policy in Africa: Evaluating the TICAD Process*, and analyzed Japan's policy toward Africa through ODA and the TICAD process over the decades.[4] Raposo published another book, *Japan's Foreign Aid to Africa: Angola and Mozambique within the TICAD Process*, observing Japan's African diplomacy through the TICAD process, especially for Angola and Mozambique as case studies.[5] In Japan, Mizuho Information & Research Institute conducted the third party evaluation research on the TICAD

---

[1] For diplomatic accomplishments by successive Japanese prime ministers, see Akimoto, Daisuke. 2022. *Japanese Prime Ministers and Their Peace Philosophy: 1945 to the Present*. Singapore: Palgrave Macmillan.

[2] Lehman, Howard. 2005. "Japan's Foreign Aid Policy to Africa Since the Tokyo International Conference on African Development". *Pacific Affairs*. Vol. 78, No. 3, pp. 423–442.

[3] Edström, Bert. 2010. "Japan and the TICAD Process". *ISDP Asia Paper*. https://isdp.eu/content/uploads/publications/2010_edstrom_japan-and-the-ticad.pdf.

[4] Amakasu Raposo, Pedro. 2014. *Japan's Foreign Aid Policy in Africa: Evaluating the TICAD Process*. New York: Palgrave.

[5] Amakasu Raposo, Pedro. 2014. *Japan's Foreign Aid to Africa: Angola and Mozambique within the TICAD Process*. New York: Routledge.

process in association with the Japanese Ministry of Foreign Affairs.[6] The earlier works have not necessarily focused on Japan's TICAD diplomacy in light of "global health" however.

Significantly, the coronavirus pandemic inevitably influenced Japan's policy toward the TICAD process, since the pandemic made global health in Africa a critical agenda item in the conference in the end. Accordingly, this chapter attempts to shed light on Japan's TICAD diplomacy for the development of Africa by contextualizing the previous TICAD initiatives in the light of human security as well as global health. It tries to explore the reason why the Japanese government has been motivated for the contributions to the African continent in terms of national interests as well as human security. This chapter clarifies the consistency of Japan's commitment to the TICAD conferences that contribute to human security and global health of Africa as well as Japan's strategic motivations to pursue its strategic foreign policy vision, namely Free and Open Indo-Pacific (FOIP) in recent years.[7]

## JAPAN'S AFRICA DIPLOMACY: TICAD CONFERENCES IN THE 1990S (TICAD 1–2)

After the end of the Cold War, the Japanese government hosted TICAD 1 in Tokyo on October 5–6, 1993, co-chaired by Parliamentary Vice-Foreign Minister Shozo Azuma.[8] On October 5, Prime Minister Morihiro Hosokawa delivered a keynote speech and argued that the Tokyo Declaration should be adopted in the conference as a guideline for the future development of Africa.[9] On the following day, the Tokyo Declaration

---

[6] Mizuho Information & Research Institute. 2017. "Evaluation of Japan's ODA to Africa through the TICAD Process for the Past 10 Years". https://www.mofa.go.jp/pol icy/oda/evaluation/FY2017/pdfs/ticad.pdf.

[7] This chapter is based on my earlier research on Japan's TICAD diplomacy. See Akimoto, Daisuke. March 31, 2022. "TICAD: The Evolution of Japan's Africa Diplomacy". *The Diplomat*. https://thediplomat.com/2022/03/ticad-the-evolution-of-japans-africa-diplomacy/.

[8] Ministry of Foreign Affairs of Japan. 1993. "List of the Participating Delegations of the Tokyo International Conference on African Development (October 5–6, 1993, Tokyo, Japan)". https://www.mofa.go.jp/region/africa/ticad/list/index.html.

[9] Ministry of Foreign Affairs of Japan. October 5, 1993. "Keynote Speech by Prime Minister Morihiro Hosokawa in TICAD". https://www.mofa.go.jp/mofaj/press/enz etsu/05/eos_1005.html.

on African Development was adopted and participants agreed on an agenda for African development, including measures against infectious diseases, which had long had a disastrous impact on the continent.[10] Thus, the TICAD initiative represents the nature of Japan's post-Cold War diplomacy toward Africa.

TICAD 2 was held by the Japanese government in cooperation with the United Nations and the Global Coalition for Africa in Tokyo on October 19–21, 1998.[11] On October 19, Prime Minister Keizo Obuchi delivered a keynote speech and contended that Japan should prioritize its contribution toward the social development of Africa, such as in primary education, water supplies, public health, and medical access.[12] On October 21, Foreign Minister Masahiko Komura stated in his policy speech at the conference that Japan would continue its support for lowering early mortality of pregnant women and infants in Africa and for addressing the HIV/AIDS epidemic and eradicating poliovirus in the continent. In addition, malaria and tuberculosis were included in the Tokyo Declaration of TICAD 2 as other main infectious diseases that should be prevented.[13] Notably, it was confirmed that Japan would cooperate with the United States on polio eradication through grassroots collaboration between the Japan Overseas Cooperation Volunteers and the United States Peace Corps.[14] In the TICAD 2 process, Obuchi as an

[10] Ministry of Foreign Affairs of Japan. October 6, 1993. "The Tokyo Declaration on African Development". https://www.mofa.go.jp/mofaj/area/ticad/tc_senge.html.

[11] Ministry of Foreign Affairs of Japan. October 19–21, 1998. "Tokyo International Conference on African Development Tokyo, October 19th-21st, 1998 List of Participants". https://www.mofa.go.jp/region/africa/ticad2/list/index.html.

[12] Ministry of Foreign Affairs of Japan. October 19, 1998. "Keynote Speech by Prime Minister Keizo Obuchi in TICAD 2". https://www.mofa.go.jp/mofaj/press/enzetsu/10/eos_1019.html.

[13] Ministry of Foreign Affairs of Japan. 1998. "The Tokyo Declaration on African Development in TICAD 2". https://www.mofa.go.jp/mofaj/area/ticad/kodo_1.html#4-1-2.

[14] Ministry of Foreign Affairs of Japan. October 21, 1998. "Japan's New Africa Support Program based on Action Plan in TICAD 2". https://www.mofa.go.jp/mofaj/area/ticad/tc_progr.html.

initiator of Japan's human security diplomacy contributed to facilitating Japan's TICAD initiative for the development of Africa.[15]

## Human Security and ODA to Africa: TICAD Conferences in the 2000s (TICAD 3–4)

After the Obuchi administration, Japan's human security diplomacy through the TICAD process was strengthened. TICAD 3 was held in Tokyo from September 29 to October 1, 2003, chaired by Yoshiro Mori as former prime minister.[16] Mori made opening remarks at the conference and stressed the importance of a concept of "human security" as one of the key visions of Japanese diplomacy.[17] After the opening remarks, a keynote speech was made by Prime Minister Junichiro Koizumi, who stated that Japan's contributions to the development of Africa should be based on the three pillars: "human-centered development, poverty reduction through economic growth, and consolidation of peace in Africa".[18] Koizumi also mentioned the concept of human security as Japan's diplomatic vision for the development of Africa under the banner of "Towards a Vibrant Africa: A Continent of Hope and Opportunity".[19]

TICAD 4 was held in Yokohama, Kanagawa Prefecture, on May 28–30, 2008, chaired by Prime Minister Yasuo Fukuda.[20] In his keynote speech, Fukuda emphasized the significance of the "maternal and child health handbook" used in Japan for maintaining the health condition of

---

[15] As for Obuchi's foreign policy on human security, see Akimoto, Daisuke. 2022. *Japanese Prime Ministers and Their Peace Philosophy: 1945 to the Present*. Singapore: Palgrave Macmillan, pp. 253–259.

[16] Ministry of Foreign Affairs of Japan. 2003. "Highlights of the Summary by the Chair of TICAD III". https://www.mofa.go.jp/region/africa/ticad3/chair-2.html.

[17] Ministry of Foreign Affairs of Japan. September 29, 2003. "Opening Remarks by Mr. Yoshiro Mori, Chairperson of TICAD III". https://www.mofa.go.jp/region/africa/ticad3/opening.html.

[18] Ministry of Foreign Affairs of Japan. September 29, 2003. "Keynote Speech by Prime Minister Junichiro Koizumi at the Third Tokyo International Conference on African Development (TICAD III)". https://www.mofa.go.jp/region/africa/ticad3/pmspeech.html.

[19] Ibid.

[20] Ministry of Foreign Affairs of Japan. May, 28–30, 2008. "The Fourth Tokyo International Conference on African Development (TICAD IV) in Yokohama 28–30 May, 2008". https://www.mofa.go.jp/region/africa/ticad/ticad4/index.html.

pregnant women and children.[21] He pointed out that a similar hand-book can be used in Africa too to promote the health of both mothers and children. Notably, Fukuda pledged that Japan would double its official development assistance (ODA) to Africa in five years. In this way, the Fukuda administration expressed its stance and contributions to achieving human security in Africa.[22]

## ABE INITIATIVE: TICAD CONFERENCES IN THE 2010S (TICAD 5–7)

TICAD 5 was held in Yokohama under the basic concept of "Hand in Hand with a More Dynamic Africa" on June 1–3, 2013, chaired by Prime Minister Shinzo Abe.[23] In his opening remarks, Abe stated that Japan would provide 650 billion yen (approximately 6.5 billion dollars) for infrastructure development in Africa in five years.[24] In the field of global health, Abe argued that the Japanese government would try to make universal health coverage (UHC) part of the "Japan brand" in the African continent. He also mentioned the role of the Japanese Self-Defense Forces in anti-piracy activities in Djibouti and nation-building operations in South Sudan to achieve human security in Africa.

[21] Ministry of Foreign Affairs of Japan. May 28, 2008. "Address by H.E. Mr. Yasuo Fukuda, Prime Minister of Japan at the Opening Session of the Fourth Tokyo International Conference on African Development (TICAD IV)". https://www.mofa.go.jp/region/africa/ticad/ticad4/pm/address.html.

[22] Ministry of Foreign Affairs of Japan. May 28–30, 2008. "Towards a Vibrant Africa. A Continent of Hope and Opportunity". https://www.mofa.go.jp/region/africa/ticad/ticad4/initiative.pdf.

[23] Ministry of Foreign Affairs of Japan. June 3, 2013. "Fifth Tokyo International Conference on African Development (TICAD V)". https://www.mofa.go.jp/region/page6e_000075.html https://www.mofa.go.jp/region/page2e_000002.html.

[24] Ministry of Foreign Affairs of Japan. June 1, 2013. "The Africa that Joins in Partnership with Japan Is Brighter Still: Address by H.E. Mr. Shinzo Abe, Prime Minister of Japan, at the Opening Session of the Fifth Tokyo International Conference on African Development (TICAD V)". https://www.mofa.go.jp/files/000005500.pdf.

During the conference, the Yokohama Declaration 2013 was adopted on June 3. The declaration emphasized the importance of infrastructure development and regional conflict prevention mechanisms.[25] In this respect, the role of the African Peace and Security Architecture should be regarded as indispensable not only for the maintenance of peace and security but also for development of Africa in general.[26] It also reconfirmed the necessity of promoting child health and supporting the African Union's Campaign for Accelerated Reduction of Maternal Mortality in Africa.[27] Japan's focus on infrastructure and conflict prevention represents its ODA diplomacy and its policy on international peacekeeping operations for Africa.

TICAD 6 was held in Nairobi, Kenya, on August 27–28, 2016, co-chaired by Abe.[28] In his keynote speech at the opening session, Abe stressed the importance of achieving UHC in Africa and touched on Japan's contribution to peacekeeping operations in the continent since 1993.[29] Notably, Abe stated that Japan "bears the responsibility of fostering the confluence of the Pacific and Indian Oceans and of Asia and Africa into a place that values freedom, the rule of law, and the market economy, free from force or coercion, and making it prosperous".[30] This statement has been regarded as the beginning of Japan's FOIP vision. It

[25] Ministry of Foreign Affairs of Japan. June 3, 2013. "Yokohama Declaration 2013: Hand in Hand with a More Dynamic Africa". https://www.mofa.go.jp/region/page3e_000053.html.

[26] African Union. 2012. "The African Peace and Security Architecture (APSA)". https://www.peaceau.org/en/topic/the-african-peace-and-security-architecture-apsa.

[27] African Union. 2020. "Campaign for Accelerated Reduction of Maternal Mortality in Africa (CARMMA) 2009–2019". https://au.int/en/pressreleases/20200206/campaign-accelerated-reduction-maternal-mortality-africa-carmma-2009-2019.

[28] Ministry of Foreign Affairs of Japan. August 28, 2016. "Sixth Tokyo International Conference on African Development (TICAD VI)". https://www.mofa.go.jp/af/af1/page3e_000551.html.

[29] Ministry of Foreign Affairs of Japan. August 27, 2016. "Address by Prime Minister Shinzo Abe at the Opening Session of the Sixth Tokyo International Conference on African Development (TICAD VI)". https://www.mofa.go.jp/afr/af2/page4e_000496.html.

[30] Ibid.

also symbolizes that Japan's African diplomacy was about to be embedded in the diplomatic vision in the long run.[31]

As an outcome of the conference, the Nairobi Declaration was adopted as agenda for sustainable development in Africa.[32] In the declaration, the establishment of a resilient health system in Africa was emphasized as one of the priorities, partially due to the outbreak of Ebola pandemic. Other communicable and non-communicable diseases, such as HIV/AIDS, tuberculosis, malaria, Zika, and yellow fever were mentioned and the importance of preventing and preparing for pandemics were stressed, as was UHC.[33] It was before the outbreak of the coronavirus pandemic, but the outbreak of the Ebola pandemic as well as the spread of infectious diseases in Africa made global health as one of the important agenda items in the TICAD 6 process.

TICAD 7 was held in Yokohama on August 28–30, 2019, chaired by Abe, and co-hosted by the United Nations, the UNDP, the World Bank, and the African Union Commission.[34] In his keynote address, Abe emphasized the fact that Japanese private investment into Africa for the past three years amounted to as much as 20 billion dollars.[35] He also stressed the significance of African Business Education Initiative for Youth (ABE Initiative) to encourage and foster young entrepreneurs in the continent.[36] During the conference, the Yokohama Declaration 2019

---

[31] Akimoto, Daisuke. 2021. "The Clash of Japan's FOIP and China's BRI?" *Journal of Politics and Development (The REST)*. Vol. 11, No. 2, pp. 88–99.

[32] Ministry of Foreign Affairs of Japan. August 26, 2016. "TICAD VI Nairobi Declaration: Advancing Africa's Sustainable Development Agenda TICAD Partnership for Prosperity". https://www.mofa.go.jp/af/af1/page3e_000543.html.

[33] Ibid.

[34] Ministry of Foreign Affairs of Japan. August 28–30, 2019. "The Seventh Tokyo International Conference on African Development (TICAD 7)". https://www.mofa.go.jp/region/africa/ticad/ticad7/index.html.

[35] Ministry of Foreign Affairs of Japan. August 28, 2019. "Keynote Address by Mr. Shinzo Abe, Prime Minister of Japan at the Opening Session of the Seventh Tokyo International Conference on African Development (TICAD 7)". https://www.mofa.go.jp/af/af1/page4e_001069.html.

[36] Ministry of Foreign Affairs of Japan. 2019. "The ABE Initiative-Pilots of African Business". https://www.mofa.go.jp/files/000469595.pdf.

was adopted on the final day.[37] The declaration acknowledged that it is imperative to promote the achievement of UHC in Africa while controlling communicable diseases, such as HIV/AIDS, tuberculosis, malaria, polio, and neglected tropical diseases (NTDs).[38] At the same time, it was confirmed that TICAD participants agreed to respect the rule of law reflected in the United Nations Convention on the Law of the Sea (UNCLOS), implying African countries' collective opposition to China's maritime policy in the South China Sea.[39] The support by the TICAD participants for the UNCLOS signifies political and strategic connotations of the TICAD process in the Indo-Pacific strategic sphere.

## The COVID-19 Period: TICAD Conference in the 2020s (TICAD 8)

On 27–28 August, 2022, TICAD 8 took place in Tunis, Tunisia and Prime Minister Fumio Kishida participated in the conference online. During the conference, Prime Minister Kishida promised that Japan would initiate "Japan's Green Growth Initiative with Africa" and invest in start-up companies by young businessmen in Japan and Africa.[40] He moreover announced that Japan would provide co-financing of up to 5 billion dollars with the African Development Bank to improve the life standard of the people in Africa, and that his administration should contribute to the public health issues in the African continent.[41] It is logical to consider that Japan's TICAD diplomacy during the Kishida administration based on the FOIP vision has been consistent with the previous administrations, but its commitment to Africa has been influenced by the outbreak of the COVID-19 pandemic.

[37] Ministry of Foreign Affairs of Japan. August 30, 2019. "Yokohama Declaration 2019. Advancing Africa's Development through People, Technology and Innovation". https://www.mofa.go.jp/region/africa/ticad/ticad7/pdf/yokohama_declaration_en.pdf.

[38] Ibid.

[39] Ibid.

[40] Prime Minister of Japan and His Cabinet. August 27, 2022. "Opening Speech by Prime Minister KISHIDA Fumio at the Opening Session of the Eighth Tokyo International Conference on African Development (TICAD 8)". https://japan.kantei.go.jp/101_kishida/statement/202208/_00017.html.

[41] Ibid.

Notably, Kishida pledged Japan's further commitment to the global health of Africa, stating that "The spread of COVID-19 has made it clear the importance of dealing with infectious diseases. I announce today that Japan will contribute up to 1.08 billion dollars to the Global Fund's Seventh Replenishment over the next three years. This is based on the idea of human security and to contribute to supporting measures against the major infectious diseases, such as HIV and AIDS, tuberculosis and malaria, and to strengthening health systems, especially in Africa". In response to the pledge, Peter Sands as CEO of the Global Fund stated that "We are extremely grateful to Prime Minister Kishida for this strong leadership and to the people of Japan for this extraordinary support to accelerate the end of HIV, tuberculosis and malaria, with a view to achieving UHC".[42]

## Japan's Motives for the Development of the African Continent

Regarding Tokyo's motivation for the development of Africa, Bolade M. Eyinla, a professor at the University of Ilorin in Nigeria, observed that Japan's policy toward TICAD has been based on its national interest.[43] In fact, it is true that the number of Japanese companies in Africa has been on the increase in recent years as shown in Fig. 5.1.[44] Moreover, the TICAD process can be seen as part of Japan's balancing diplomacy against the rise of China, as pointed out by Kyoto University Professor Motoki Takahashi.[45] Given Abe's keynote speech at TICAD 6, it is fair to analyze that the TICAD process has been embedded in Japan's FOIP vision vis-à-vis China's Belt and Road Initiative, and hence, it is possible

[42] The Global Fund. August 27, 2022. "Global Fund Applauds Japan's Major Commitment to Help End AIDS, Tuberculosis and Malaria and Strengthen Systems for Health". https://www.theglobalfund.org/en/news/2022/2022-08-27-global-fund-app lauds-japans-major-commitment-to-help-end-aids-tuberculosis-and-malaria-and-strengthen-systems-for-health/.

[43] Eyinla, Bolade M. 2018. "Promoting Japan's National Interest in Africa". *African Development*. Vol. 43, No. 3, pp. 107–122.

[44] Japan Times. August 26, 2022. "Prospects Bright as Investment Climbs". https://www.japantimes.co.jp/2022/08/26/special-supplements/prospects-bright-investment-climbs/.

[45] Takahashi, Motoki. 2017. "Changes in TICADs and the World: The Role of Japan in African Development Reconsidered". *Africa Report*. No. 55, pp. 47–61.

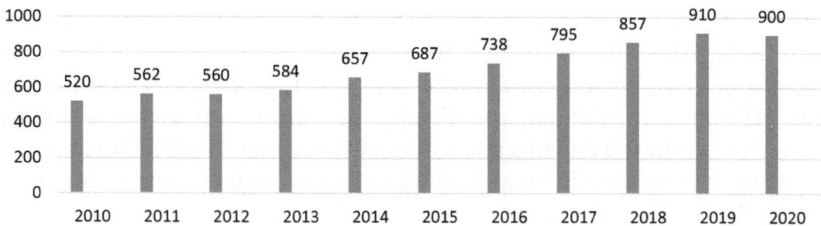

**Fig. 5.1** The number of Japanese corporate offices in Africa 2010–2020 (*Note* Created by the author based on data by Japan Times on August 26, 2022)

to argue that Japan's commitment to the development of Africa has been in Japan's national interests.

It is an undeniable fact that Japanese companies have been in competition with Chinese counterparts in the African continent. While Japan has been committed to the development of Africa, China has made considerable contributions to the infrastructure and "aggressive selling of a variety of goods".[46] According to a survey conducted by the Japan External Trade Organization to Japanese businesses in Africa in 2018, 22.9 percent of Japanese firms replied that Chinese companies are major rivals in the continent. The survey result regarding the competing firms in Africa is: (1) Chinese companies (22.9 percent), (2) European companies (21.6 percent), Japanese companies (18.9 percent), local companies (12 percent), and American companies (7.6 percent), although Chinese companies are potential partners for Japanese firms at the same time.[47]

Having said that, it needs to be noted that the amount of Japan's foreign direct investment fell from 2013 to 2020,[48] and hence, Japan's contributions to the development of Africa are not necessarily based on business and investment purposes. If anything, a re-examination of the previous TICAD conferences, keynote speeches, and declarations in this chapter indicates that Japan's TICAD diplomacy has been based not only

[46] Shinozaki, Natsuki. September 6, 2019. "Japan and China in Africa: From Competition to Collaboration". *NHK News*. https://www3.nhk.or.jp/nhkworld/en/news/backstories/662/.

[47] Ibid.

[48] African Development Bank. August 26, 2022. "Abe's Legacy in Africa under Scrutiny at Development Summit". https://www.afdb.org/en/news-and-events/abes-legacy-africa-under-scrutiny-development-summit-54367.

on its national interests, but also on humanitarian purposes, i.e., human security for the African people. In particular, public health and disease prevention have been consistent themes since TICAD 1 in 1993. During the TICAD 8 in Tunisia, the Kishida administration pledged further contributions to the enhancement of basic human needs and human security in the African continent as it continues to struggle for recovering from the COVID-19 pandemic.

## CONCLUSION

This chapter has examined Japan's contributions to the development of Africa through its diplomatic contributions to TICAD conferences. Throughout the diplomatic initiative, the Japanese government has contributed to the development in Africa including global health issues, including the spread of maternal and child health handbook in the African continent. Japan's TICAD diplomacy has shown that its contributions to global health issues, such as the three major infectious diseases (HIV/AIDS, tuberculosis, malaria), NTDs, and poliovirus, have been consistent throughout its human security diplomacy toward Africa. It has been confirmed that the Japanese government has made consistent contributions to the development of Africa since 1993. Furthermore, it has been confirmed that Japan's TICAD diplomacy has contributed to enhancing global health in Africa especially during the COVID-19 pandemic period.

As for motivations of the Japanese government, it has been observed that Japan's Africa diplomacy has been based on the FOIP vision, and therefore, has been influenced by the strategic competition with China's Belt and Road Initiative. Without a doubt, Japan's contributions to the development of Africa have been motivated by its national interests, and the number of Japanese companies in Africa has been on the increase in recent years as discussed. Nevertheless, it has been also clarified that Japan's commitments to the TICAD processes have been based on its human security policy as well as humanitarian purposes for global health, especially after the outbreak of the COVID-19 pandemic. The Japanese government announced that TICAD 9 would be held in Yokohama in 2025.[49] Based on its human security concept as its diplomatic pillar as

---

[49] Ministry of Foreign Affairs of Japan. August 8, 2023. "Decision on the Host City of Ninth Tokyo International Conference on African Development (TICAD 9)". https://www.mofa.go.jp/press/release/press7e_000026.html.

well as Kishida's "new capitalism" investing in "human capital" and "people" in Japan, Africa, and around the globe,[50] Japan is expected to make further diplomatic contributions to the development as well as global health of the African continent.

[50] Kato, Kazuyo. August 29, 2022. "Kishida Shows Leadership at TICAD on Global Health and Security". *Japan Times*. https://www.japantimes.co.jp/opinion/2022/08/29/commentary/japan-commentary/japan-ticad-pledge/.

# CHAPTER 6

# Japan's Changing ODA Diplomacy for Global Health

**Abstract** Japan's policy on official development assistance (ODA) has been changing over time. In essence, Japan's ODA strategy has been conditioned by global politics. In the postwar period, it was related to Tokyo's postwar reparation, and was influenced by the Cold War politics afterwards. In the post-Cold War era, Japan became the top ODA donor, and recently, the ODA policy has been embedded in its diplomatic vision, namely the Free and Open Indo-Pacific (FOIP). Does Japan's foreign policy undergo a paradigm shift in its ODA diplomacy for global health in the coronavirus pandemic world? This chapter sheds light on the development of Japan's ODA policy and its implications for Japan's global health policy in the COVID-19 world.

**Keywords** Development Cooperation Charter · Global health · Japan · ODA Charter · Official development assistance (ODA)

## INTRODUCTION

Japan's policy on official development assistance (ODA) has been changing over time. In March 2022 for instance, Japan's ODA to China was completely terminated. Japan's ODA to China began in December 1979, when former Prime Minister Masayoshi Ohira visited Beijing. In

© The Author(s), under exclusive license to Springer Nature Singapore Pte Ltd. 2024
D. Akimoto, *Japan and Global Health*,
https://doi.org/10.1007/978-981-97-0972-4_6

total, Japan's ODA to China amounted to 3.65 trillion yen in loan aid, while promoting 231 projects related to the establishment of basic infrastructure.[1] Chinese Premier Zhou Enlai had decided to give up on pressing Japan for war reparations, stating in a meeting with Foreign Minister Takeo Miki in April 21, 1972, "It is true that Chinese people are the victims of Japanese militarism, but Japanese people are also actually the victims. We cannot accept the compensation because it is immoral".[2] In this sense, it can be argued that Japan's ODA to China played an indispensable role in the bilateral reconciliation process in place of war reparations.

The termination of Japan's ODA to China was announced by Prime Minister Shinzo Abe in 2018. Now that China is the world's second largest economy, dwarfing the Japanese economy, it seemed only natural for Tokyo to terminate its ODA to China. Beijing itself is now a supplier of economic assistance and has promoted its Belt and Road Initiative to build infrastructure overseas. At the same time, it was thought to be strategically imperative for Tokyo to end ODA to China in the middle of the China-US economic and geopolitical competition in the Indo-Pacific. *Sankei Shimbun* reported the end of Japan's ODA to China as the "end of a momentous foreign policy failure".[3] Japan's economic assistance, especially grant aid for global health, has been redirected to Southeast Asia, South America, and Africa.[4]

In essence, Japan's ODA strategy was conditioned by global politics. In the postwar period, it was related to Tokyo's postwar reparation, and was influenced by the Cold War politics afterwards. In the post-Cold War era, Japan became the top ODA donor, and more recently, the ODA policy has been embedded in its diplomatic vision, namely the Free and Open

---

[1] Nippon.com. November 6, 2018. "After 40 Years, Japan Stops Aid to China". https://www.nippon.com/en/features/h00321/.

[2] Xu, Xianfen. 2013. "Japan's Official Development Assistance (ODA) Policy towards China: The Role of Emotional Factors". *Journal of Contemporary East Asia Studies*. Vol. 2, No. 1, pp. 77–94.

[3] Komori, Yoshihisa. November 8, 2018. "Japan's ODA to China: End of a Momentous Foreign Policy Failure". *Japan Forward*. https://japan-forward.com/japans-oda-to-china-end-of-a-momentous-foreign-policy-failure/.

[4] Nikkei Shimbun. August 21, 2021. "Japan's ODA, Highest Record in Its History". https://www.nikkei.com/article/DGKKZO74392650R00C21A8PE8000/.

Indo-Pacific (FOIP) concept as pointed out by Japan Business Federation (Keidanren).[5] Does the end of Japan's ODA to China signify Japan's foreign policy shift in its ODA diplomacy in the Indo-Pacific region? Or does Japan's foreign policy undergo a paradigm shift in its ODA diplomacy for global health toward the post-COVID world?[6] This chapter sheds light on the development of Japan's ODA policy and its implications for Japan's global health policy in the COVID-19 world.[7]

## Historical Background
## of Japan's Changing ODA Policy

Historically, Japan's ODA policy was developed in the process of its post-war economic recovery and reintegration as a member state of the international community. Based on the recognition that the restrictions on trade after the Great Depression led to the prolonged recession that eventually caused World War II, the Bretton Woods Agreements were signed in July 1944. In this context, the International Monetary Fund (IMF), the General Agreement on Tariffs and Trade (GATT), and the International Bank for Reconstruction and Development (IBRD) were established with a view to stabilizing the world economy and making financial contributions to reconstruction of war-damaged countries as well as developing countries. Japan's rapid economic growth in the post-war period owed to the financial assistance and free trade system of these international organizations.

In the process of its postwar economic recovery and reconstruction however, Japan stopped being an aid recipient, and started supporting developing countries in Asia in the middle of the Cold War. Japan signed

[5] Keidanren. March 11, 2021. "Exchange Opinions on the Current Situation and the Future Agenda of ODA". http://www.keidanren.or.jp/journal/times/2021/0311_05.html.

[6] Japan Center for International Exchange (JCIE). 2021. "Japan's Global Health Diplomacy in the Post-COVID Era: The Paradigm Shift Needed on ODA and Related Policies". https://www.jcie.org/wp-content/uploads/2021/03/Full-DAH-report-final-web.pdf.

[7] This chapter is based on my earlier research on Japan's ODA diplomacy in terms of global health. See Akimoto, Daisuke. February 10, 2022. "Japan's Changing ODA Diplomacy". The Diplomat. https://thediplomat.com/2022/02/japans-changing-oda-diplomacy/.

the Colombo Plan in 1954,[8] began its ODA diplomacy to countries mainly in the Asia–Pacific region, and eventually became the world's largest ODA donor in 1989, surpassing the United States. From 1991 to 2000, Japan was the world's largest ODA supplier.[9] Since 2001, the United States has retaken the top spot, but Japan has remained one of the major ODA donors as a member state of the Development Assistance Committee (DAC) of the Organization for Economic Cooperation and Development (OECD). Therefore, it can be observed that Japan's ODA policy has been shaped and conditioned based on national interests, its economic power, and the ideal of international cooperation as reflected in the ODA Charter.

## The Development of Japan's ODA Charter

Japan's first ODA Charter was created based on a cabinet decision in June 1992.[10] The philosophical elements of the charter are: (1) "humanitarian considerations, (2) recognition of the interdependent relationships in the international community, (3) the necessity of conservation of the environment, and (4) the necessity of supporting self-help efforts by developing countries".[11] The 1992 ODA Charter paid attention to environmental protection, the non-military purpose of aid and the military expenditure of recipients, and recipient states' accomplishments in establishing a market-oriented economic system, democracy, human rights, and freedom.[12] Again, it needs to be noted that Japan's ODA diplomacy was conditioned by its policy on war reparations as well as the political context of the Cold War.

---

[8] Colombo Plan. 2022. "The Colombo Plan". https://colombo-plan.org.

[9] Japan International Cooperation Agency (JICA). 2022. "About ODA in the World". https://www.jica.go.jp/aboutoda/basic/05.html.

[10] Ministry of Foreign Affairs of Japan. 1997. "Japan's ODA Charter". https://www.mofa.go.jp/policy/oda/summary/1997/09.html.

[11] Ibid.

[12] Ibid.

Japan's ODA Charter was revised in 2003,[13] with a view to stipulating the significance of "national interests" in its ODA policy.[14] The four basic philosophical elements were not changed, but the revised ODA Charter focused on (1) "support for self-help efforts of developing countries, (2) importance of the human security concept, (3) assurances of fairness, (4) utilization of Japan's experience and expertise, and (5) cooperation in the international community".[15] Specifically, it raised the following priorities: "poverty reduction, sustainable economic growth, peacebuilding, and the United Nations Millennium Development Goals (MDGs)".[16] Thus, although it stressed the significance of human security and international cooperation, the revision of Japan's ODA Charter reflected realistic perspectives on Japan's policy toward international cooperation based on the significance of national interests.

In March 2014, Foreign Minister Fumio Kishida announced an official plan to revise the ODA Charter, stating, "As we move into a new era, ODA that has built up a 60-year history must also evolve. In this light, I have decided this year to review and revise the ODA Charter".[17] In 2015, the Japanese government decided to change the name of the ODA Charter to the Development Cooperation Charter. The Development Cooperation Charter was drafted based on a cabinet decision of February 2015.[18] Notably, the Development Cooperation Charter enables the Japanese government to provide foreign military forces with assistance for non-military purposes, such as humanitarian activities. The Japanese government explained that the revised Charter was not designed

---

[13] Ministry of Foreign Affairs of Japan. 2013. "Japan's Official Development Assistance Charter". https://www.mofa.go.jp/policy/oda/reform/revision0308.pdf.

[14] Sunaga, Kazuto. 2004. "The Reshaping of Japan's Official Development Assistance (ODA) Charter". *Discussion Paper on Development Assistance*. No. 3, pp. 1–31.

[15] Ministry of Foreign Affairs of Japan. March 14, 2013. "Review of Japan's Official Development Assistance Charter". https://www.mofa.go.jp/policy/oda/reform/review0303.html.

[16] Ibid.

[17] Ministry of Foreign Affairs of Japan. 2015. "Decision on Development Cooperation Charter". https://www.mofa.go.jp/files/000067702.pdf.

[18] Ministry of Foreign Affairs of Japan. February 10, 2015. "Cabinet Decision on the Development Cooperation Charter". https://www.mofa.go.jp/mofaj/gaiko/oda/files/000067701.pdf.

to contribute to the prolonging of any conflicts.[19] At the same time, the Japanese government attempted to legitimatize its ODA diplomacy by featuring an animated character called "ODA-man".[20]

Writing for *The Diplomat*, Ankit Panda observed that Japan's ODA policy is consistent with a "mercantile realist approach" to international affairs and that the revised Charter includes "non-combat military aid".[21] For example, as part of its ODA diplomacy Japan provided military bands of Papua New Guinea with musical instruments in 2017. Japan moreover provided life-saving equipment used by the Self-Defense Forces in rescue missions during natural disasters to the Philippine military.[22] Either way, Japan's ODA policy was influenced by Japan's security policy based on its national interests as well as the changing security environment surrounding Japan.

## Japan's ODA Budget and the Revision of the Development Cooperation Charter during the COVID-19 Pandemic

In December 2021, Finance Minister Shunichi Suzuki and Foreign Minister Yoshimasa Hayashi decided to increase the amount of Japan's ODA for Fiscal Year 2022, a budget move related to Japan's FOIP vision.[23] This decision was made and facilitated by the ruling Liberal Democratic Party (LDP) against opposition from the Ministry of Finance, which had pointed out that there were still some remaining funds inside

---

[19] Ministry of Foreign Affairs of Japan. March 8, 2015. "Rebuttal Statement against the Editorial of *Japan Times*: 'Aid That Could Foment Conflict' (February 20, 2015)". https://www.mofa.go.jp/policy/oda/page_000139.html.

[20] Lindgren, Wrenn Yennie. 2020. "WIN–WIN! with ODA-man: Legitimizing Development Assistance Policy in Japan". *Pacific Review*. Vol. 34, No. 4, pp. 633–663.

[21] Panda, Ankit. February 9, 2015. "Japan to Open Military Aid Channel". *The Diplomat*. https://thediplomat.com/2015/02/japan-to-open-military-aid-channel/.

[22] Sato, Tatsuya and Naoki Matsuyama. April 20, 2021. "SDF Helping Army in Philippines in ODA Context". *Asahi Shimbun*. https://www.asahi.com/ajw/articles/14334087.

[23] Mainichi. December 24, 2021. "Grant Aid ODA to Be Slightly Increased by LDP's Support, Outnegotiating the Finance Ministry". https://mainichi.jp/articles/20211224/k00/00m/010/273000c.

the Japan International Cooperation Agency (JICA).[24] In other words, the FOIP vision was regarded as an important factor to increase the amount of Japan's ODA budget so that Japan would be able to compete with China's Belt and Road Initiative which has been increasing its political influence around the world.

Meanwhile, it can be observed that the Kishida administration has attempted to increase ODA budget as a tool for Japanese diplomacy.[25] During the Eighth Tokyo International Conference on African Development (TICAD 8) held in Tunisia, Kishida promised to make a proactive contribution to enhancing the global health system in order to curb the spread of COVID-19. Japan's ODA diplomacy, therefore, is undergoing a policy transformation to include further contributions to global health, as well as for the facilitation of the FOIP vision vis-à-vis China's Belt and Road Initiative. Japan's ODA has tended to focus on energy and infrastructure rather than global health and nutrition, but in the midst of the coronavirus pandemic, the Japanese government is expected to increase its ODA budget for global health and nutrition.[26]

In the meanwhile, the Kishida government revised Japan's National Security Strategy on December 16, 2022. Japan's ODA policy has "strong affinity" with the National Security Strategy, and the nature of Japan's ODA has been increasingly linked with international security issues.[27] Following the revision of the National Security Strategy, the Development Cooperation Charter was revised in June 2023 in order to promote its FOIP vision in the Indo-Pacific region.[28] Indeed, the 2022 National Security Strategy emphasized the importance of the strategic use of ODA from the perspective of Japan's FOIP vision, stipulating that "Japan

---

[24] Ibid.

[25] Japan Times. June 20, 2022. "Japan Seeking to Increase ODA Budget to Support Kishida's Diplomacy Vision". https://www.japantimes.co.jp/news/2022/06/20/national/increase-oda-budget-kishida/.

[26] As for Japan's contribution to global health ODA, see Nomura, Shuhei, Lisa Yamasaki, Kazuki Shimizu, Cyrus Ghaznavi, and Haruka Sakamoto. 2022. "Japan's Development Assistance for Health: Historical Trends and Prospects for a New Era". *Lancet*. Vol. 22, No. 100403, pp. 1–9.

[27] Nishida, Ippeita. August 10, 2022. "Revising the Development Cooperation Charter: Issues in Linking ODA and Security". Sasakawa Peace Foundation: International Information Network Analysis. https://www.spf.org/iina/en/articles/nishida_02.html.

[28] Nen, Satomi. September 7, 2022. "Japan to Review ODA Policy to Strengthen Indo-Pacific Ties". *Asahi Shimbun*. https://www.asahi.com/ajw/articles/14713027.

will strategically utilize ODA to maintain and develop a free and open international order and to realize coexistence and coprosperity in the international community".[29] The new National Security Strategy moreover confirmed the importance of "human security", noting that "under the concept of 'human security', Japan will lead international efforts to solve global issues such as poverty reduction, health, climate change, environment, and humanitarian assistance".[30]

Thus, Japan's ODA strategy has both strategic and humanitarian elements, representing both realist and liberalist perspectives (national and international interests). Given the FOIP vision and a China factor, it can be argued that Japan's ODA policy has been influenced and shaped by the changing international security environment. At the same time however, the coronavirus pandemic became a turning-point for Japan's ODA policy toward global health, which was inevitably reflected in the new Development Cooperation Charter revised in June 2023.[31]

Indeed, the 2023 Development Cooperation Charter emphasized the significance of global health, noting that: "Japan will contribute to developing global health architecture, strengthen prevention, preparedness, and responses for future public health emergencies, and promote more resilient, more equitable, and more sustainable universal health coverage (UHC) through strengthening health systems in developing countries, including the development of human resources for health"[32] based on the 2022 Global Health Strategy. It reiterates the importance of Japan's contribution to global health, stipulating that: "Japan will contribute more actively to rulemaking in fields such as global health and the environment".[33]

As a result of the COVID-19 pandemic, moreover, Japan's ODA diplomacy has been faced with the necessity of further policy readjustment. As recommended in the report by the Japan Center for International

---

[29] Ministry of Foreign Affairs of Japan. December 16, 2022. "National Security Strategy of Japan" (Provisional Translation), p. 17. https://www.cas.go.jp/jp/siryou/221216anz enhoshou/nss-e.pdf.

[30] Ibid.

[31] Ministry of Foreign Affairs of Japan. October 10, 2023. "Development Cooperation Charter: Japan's Contributions to the Sustainable Development of a Free and Open World". https://www.mofa.go.jp/mofaj/gaiko/oda/files/100514705.pdf.

[32] Ibid., p. 10.

[33] Ibid., p. 11.

Exchange,[34] it is fair to argue that it is necessary for Japan's ODA policy to prioritize economic assistance for global health, especially international cooperation for the current and future pandemics within the framework of the COVAX Facility, Gavi, the Vaccine Alliance, and the Coalition for Epidemic Preparedness Innovations (CEPI).

As shown in Fig. 6.1, 20.2 percent of respondents answered that Japan's health ODA should be increased, whereas 64.5 percent replied that the amount should be kept the same as it is now, according to a public opinion survey conducted by the Health and Global Policy Institute on August 22, 2022.[35] The result of the public opinion survey indicates that it would be significant for those who wish to increase Japan's global health ODA to advocate for the paradigm shift of Japan's ODA policy for the sake of global health security. In this sense, it is fair to argue that the outbreak of the coronavirus provided an opportunity for the changing Japan's ODA strategy in the pandemic world.

## CONCLUSION

This chapter has examined Japan's ODA policy in relation with global health in the pre-and post-COVID-19 pandemic. First, it was discussed that Japan's ODA toward China was terminated in March 2022. It was confirmed that Japan's ODA diplomacy has been motivated by national interests. Indeed, Japan's ODA was utilized as a diplomatic tool for postwar reconciliation and reparation during the Cold War period. In the post-Cold War period, Japan's ODA Charter was created with some philosophical elements in 1992. In 2003, the ODA Chater was revised taking both national interests and the MDGs into consideration. In 2015, the Development Cooperation Charter replaced the previous ODA Charter, including official assistance for non-military purposes to foreign military forces that could contribute to humanitarian assistance. In the meanwhile, the Japanese government has strengthened its public diplomacy on its ODA strategy through the creation of the ODA-man.

---

[34] Japan Center for International Exchange (JCIE). 2021. "Japan's Global Health Diplomacy in the Post-COVID Era: The Paradigm Shift Needed on ODA and Related Policies". https://www.jcie.org/wp-content/uploads/2021/03/Full-DAH-report-final-web.pdf.

[35] Health and Global Policy Institute (HGPI). August 22, 2022. "The Public Opinion Survey on Global Health". https://hgpi.org/en/research/gh-survey202208.html.

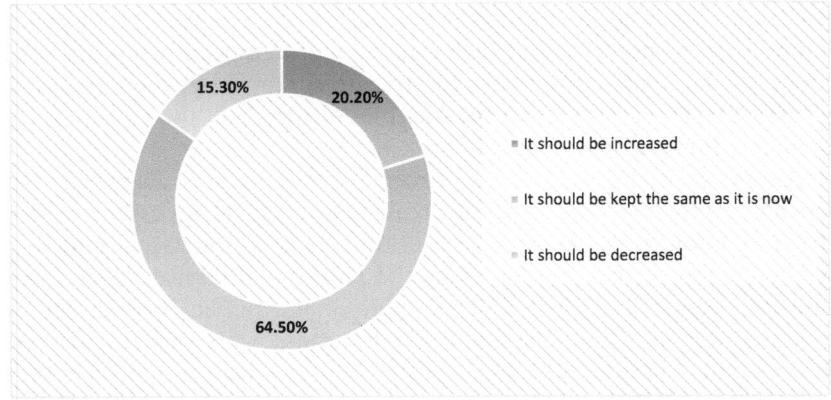

**Fig. 6.1** Poll on the proportion of ODA contributions that should be devoted to health sector (*Note N* = 1000. FY 2021 Public Opinion Survey by the Health and Global Policy Institute)

In June 2023, the Development Cooperation Charter was revised and global health was incorporated as one of the key elements of Japan's ODA policy. Japan's ODA policy has been focused on energy and infrastructure, but it has to be shifted to the field of global health in response to the current pandemic, and in preparation for the future pandemic as well. It has been also discussed that it would be necessary for those who wish to increase Japan's global health ODA, like Japanese Business Leaders' Coalition for Global Health to be examined in the next chapter, to conduct nationwide advocacy to change the mindset of the Japanese public. The paradigm shift in Japan's ODA policy will be of significance in securing the necessary budget for global health in developing countries in the middle of the pandemic period and as a way of preventing and preparing for the next pandemic.

# CHAPTER 7

# Japan and the Business Leaders' Coalition for Global Health

**Abstract** The Japanese government has facilitated global health policy and it formulated Japan's Global Health Strategy on May 24, 2022. On December 3, 2021, Bill Gates and Prime Minister Fumio Kishida held a teleconference during which they agreed that the Bill & Melinda Gates Foundation (Gates Foundation) and the Japanese government would collaborate to cope with the COVID-19 pandemic and to support a summit on the global challenge of malnutrition in Tokyo. The details of the teleconference were not broadcast, but what did the billionaire philanthropist discuss with the Japanese prime minister? This chapter examines the role of the Gates Foundation as well as the Japanese "Business Leaders' Coalition for Global Health" as part of stakeholders and promotors of global health policy in Japan and the world.

**Keywords** Bill & Melinda Gates Foundation (Gates Foundation) · Business Leaders' Coalition for Global Health · Global Health Academy · Global Health Action Japan · Global Health Strategy

## Introduction

Since its inception, the Kishida government has facilitated global health policy and it formulated Japan's Global Health Strategy on May 24, 2022.[1] A midterm plan of the strategy was drafted and submitted to a conference of the Cabinet on December 22, 2021. Meanwhile, on December 3, 2021, Bill Gates and Prime Minister Fumio Kishida held a teleconference during which they agreed that the Bill & Melinda Gates Foundation (Gates Foundation) and the Japanese government would collaborate to cope with the COVID-19 pandemic and to support a summit on the global challenge of malnutrition in Tokyo.

In Japan, the image of Bill Gates is dominated by his status as the billionaire founder of Microsoft, but it is not necessarily widely recognized that he is an active philanthropist who has worked for the enhancement of global health and nutrition conditions in developing countries. The details of the teleconference were not broadcast, but what did the billionaire philanthropist discuss with the Japanese prime minister? This chapter examines the role of the Gates Foundation as well as the Japanese "Business Leaders' Coalition for Global Health" as part of stakeholders and promotors of global health policy in Japan and the world.[2]

## The Gates-Kishida Talks and the Tokyo Nutrition for Growth Summit 2021

On December 7, 2021, the Tokyo Nutrition for Growth Summit was hosted by the Japanese government.[3] Notably, international political leaders from about 30 countries, such as Félix Antoine Tshisekedi Tshilombo (president of Congo), Sheikh Hasina (prime minister of Bangladesh), Taur Matan Ruak (prime minister of Timor-Leste), heads

---

[1] Akimoto, Daisuke. September 21, 2022. "Japan's Global Health Strategy: A Diplomatic Foresight on the G7 Hiroshima Summit". *ISDP Voices*. https://isdp.eu/japans-global-health-strategy-a-diplomatic-foresight-on-the-g7-hiroshima-summit/.

[2] This chapter is based on my earlier research on the Japanese Business Leaders' Coalition for Global Health. See Akimoto, Daisuke. December 28, 2021. "The Gates-Kishida Talks and Japan's New 'Global Health Strategy'". *The Diplomat*. https://thediplomat.com/2021/12/the-gates-kishida-talks-and-japans-new-global-health-strategy/.

[3] Ministry of Foreign Affairs of Japan. August 4, 2022. "Results Overview of the Tokyo Nutrition for Growth (N4G) Summit 2021 (Day 1: High Level Sessions)". https://www.mofa.go.jp/ic/ghp/page6e_000264.html.

of international organizations, such as António Guterres (United Nations secretary-general), David R. Malpass (president of the World Bank Group), Tedros Adhanom Ghebreyesus (director general of the World Health Organization: WHO), and representatives from civil society organizations, including the Gates Foundation, participated in the summit with a view to tackling global nutritional problems aggravated by the coronavirus pandemic.

In the opening speech of the summit, Kishida stated that Japan would make a financial contribution of 1 billion dollars to the COVAX Facility, donate approximately 10 million doses of COVID-19 vaccines to Africa, and work for combating omicron, a new variant of the coronavirus.[4] Thus, it can be observed that Kishida's announcement for Japan's international cooperation for the combat of COVID-19 as well as the improvement of global health and nutrition was encouraged and facilitated by international organizations and non-governmental organizations, including the Gates Foundation. Given the earlier Gates-Kishida talks, it is fair to argue that Bill Gates has been influential in the development of Japan's global health policy. This was not the first time that Gates and the Gates Foundation had requested the Japanese government to expand its contribution to global health and nutrition issues as discussed in the following section.

## The Role of the Bill & Melinda Gates Foundation for Global Health

Previously, Bill Gates held a telephone conference with Prime Minister Yoshihide Suga on January 12, 2021.[5] In the conference, Gates expressed his appreciation for Japan's financial contribution to Gavi, the Vaccine Alliance, and Suga showed his respect for the Gates Foundation's contribution to the enhancement of global health situation, and emphasized Japan's consistent commitment to facilitating the achievement of universal health coverage (UHC) based on "human security" as Japan's diplomatic

---

[4] Ministry of Foreign Affairs of Japan. 2021. "Opening Speech by Prime Minister, Mr. Kishida at the Tokyo Nutrition for Growth (N4G) Summit 2021". https://www.mofa.go.jp/files/100269401.pdf

[5] Ministry of Foreign Affairs of Japan. January 12, 2021. "Telephone Talk between Prime Minister SUGA Yoshihide and Co-Chair of the Bill & Melinda Gates Foundation Bill Gates". https://www.mofa.go.jp/ic/ghp/page4e_001109.html.

principle. Both Gates and Suga agreed that sufficient supply of vaccines was necessary for the combat of the coronavirus and the success of the Tokyo Olympics.[6]

In addition, the Gates Foundation has strenuously collaborated with Japanese business leaders for global health and handed out a request form to Prime Minister Suga in cooperation with the Business Leaders' Coalition for Global Health on April 27, 2021.[7] The coalition was represented by Ken Shibusawa, chief executive officer (CEO) of Shibusawa & Company, a descendant of Eiichi Shibusawa, who made a significant contribution to the formation of modern capitalism in Japan. Although the representative of the coalition was Shibusawa, the Gates Foundation successfully coordinated with influential Japanese companies, such as Sysmex, Shionogi, Toyota Tsusho, Daiwa Securities, miup, Sumitomo Chemical, NEC, Suntory, Yamaha Motor, SORA Technology, and Saraya.

## THE ROLE OF JAPANESE BUSINESS LEADERS' COALITION FOR GLOBAL HEALTH

Japanese companies have sought to make medical and pharmaceutical contributions toward the amelioration of global health conditions. Shionogi has developed effective vaccines against coronavirus including the omicron variant.[8] In the field of global health, Shionogi has worked with World Vision for reduction of the child and maternal mortality of Kenya since 2015. Based on donations from Shionogi employees as a fund source, Shionogi's "Mother to Mother Project" has contributed to improving the environment of pregnancy and childbirth by reducing the risk of infectious diseases in sub-Saharan Africa.[9]

---

[6] Japan Times. January 12, 2021. "Suga and Gates Say Vaccines for Developing Countries Key for Olympics". https://www.japantimes.co.jp/news/2021/01/12/national/suga-gates-vaccines-developing-countries-olympics/.

[7] Mitsubishi UFJ Research and Consulting. 2021. "Global Health Business Leader Coalition Handed out a Request Form to PM Suga". https://www.digitalsociety.murc.jp/globalhealth/architecture/policy/20210427_coalition_en/index.html.

[8] Nikkei Asia. November 30, 2021. "Shionogi and Daiichi Sankyo Join Hunt for Omicron Vaccine". https://asia.nikkei.com/Spotlight/Coronavirus/COVID-vaccines/Shionogi-and-Daiichi-Sankyo-join-hunt-for-omicron-vaccine.

[9] Shionogi. 2022. "Mother to Mother SHIONOGI Project". https://www.shionogi.com/global/en/sustainability/society/social-contribution-activities/mtom.html.

As a means of conveying medicines and vaccines in developing countries, Toyota Tsusho developed refrigerated vaccine transport vehicles to promote vaccine access.[10] In March 2021, Toyota's vaccine transport land cruisers obtained the world's first authentication for performance, quality, and safety prequalification for medical devices and equipment set by the WHO. Toyota Tsusho delivered vaccine transport vehicles to African countries, such as Ghana.[11] SORA Technology has worked for improving medical and health infrastructure by utilizing drones and flying vehicles for the purpose of facilitating the realization of UHC.[12]

Japanese companies have also made technological contributions to the global health field. NEC has succeeded in applying its fingerprint authentication system to the world's first child fingerprint identification solution to assist in boosting essential medication and immunization in developing countries.[13] Notably, fingerprint identification collaboratively developed by Simprints could be applied to immunization certificates for COVID-19 vaccinations in the middle of the coronavirus pandemic.[14] By applying artificial intelligence (AI) and information and communication technology (ICT) to health check-up and medical treatment, miup has been committed to the facilitation of efficient medical access and inexpensive healthcare service in Bangladesh.[15]

Based on their corporate social responsibility, some Japanese companies have attempted to contribute to eradicating lethal infectious diseases, especially malaria. For instance, Sumitomo Chemical developed insecticide-treated mosquito net (*kaya*), Olyset Net, for the purpose of

---

[10] Toyota Tsusho. December 17, 2021. "Toyota Tsusho Delivers First Refrigerated Vaccine Transport Vehicles to the Ghana Ministry of Health". https://www.toyota-tsusho.com/english/press/detail/211217_005879.html.

[11] Ibid.

[12] SORA Technology. 2022. "About Us". https://www.toyota-tsusho.com/english/press/detail/211217_005879.html.

[13] NEC. June 6, 2019 "Gavi, NEC, and Simprints to Deploy World's First Scalable Child Fingerprint Identification Solution to Boost Immunization in Developing Countries". https://www.nec.com/en/press/201906/global_20190606_01.html.

[14] Subramanian, Samantha. August 13, 2020. "Biometric Tracking Can Ensure Billions Have Immunity Against Covid-19". *Bloomberg*. https://www.bloomberg.com/features/2020-covid-vaccine-tracking-biometric/.

[15] miup. 2022. "About Us". https://miup.jp/aboutus/.

reducing and eliminating malaria in the world.[16] The Olyset Net, as a long-lasting insecticidal net, is the world's first mosquito net endorsed by the WHO, and it has been supplied to more than 100 countries through international organizations, such as the United Nations Children's Fund (UNICEF). Likewise, Sysmex has been dedicated to reducing and eliminating infectious diseases by promoting its diagnostic techniques in hematology for early detection and treatment.[17]

In order to help enhance basic hygiene in developing countries, Saraya initiated a project called "Wash a Million Hands" in Uganda in 2010 in order to promote a hand-washing culture with soap to prevent infectious diseases, such as cholera from spreading among the people in Africa.[18] Moreover, the company launched "Saraya Safe Motherhood Project" in 2018 to propagate alcohol disinfectant for safe childbirth at hospitals and maternity centers. Similarly, Yamaha Motor has contributed to public health in Africa and Asia by its "clean water supply system".[19] By introducing the original water purification system for clean drinking water, it has been reported that sanitation, health conditions, and lifestyles of the people in installed countries have been drastically improved.

In order to procure sustainable financial support for global health, Daiwa Securities has made a financial contribution to the global supply of vaccines within the framework of the International Finance Facility for Immunization Company (IFFIm) in affiliation with Gavi and the World Bank.[20] Daiwa Securities has issued vaccine bonds for Japanese investors in support of child immunization program. Moreover, Suntory, a major Japanese beverage company, has made financial

[16] Sumitomo Chemical. 2022. "Sumitomo Chemical's Initiatives to Counter Malaria". https://www.sumitomo-chem.co.jp/english/sustainability/social_contributions/olyset net/initiative/.

[17] Sysmex. April 26, 2021. "Dedicated to Eliminating Malaria through the Development of Diagnostic Devices". https://www.sysmex.co.jp/en/stories/210426_02.html.

[18] Japan Times. April 27, 2019. "Improving Health Practices through a Hands-on Approach". https://www.japantimes.co.jp/2019/08/27/special-supplements/improving-health-practices-hands-approach/.

[19] United Nations Industrial Development Organization (UNIDO). 2022. "YAMAHA Clean Water Supply System Improves People's Lives in Rural Areas". http://www.unido.or.jp/en/technology_db/1674/.

[20] Daiwa Securities Group. 2020. "Daiwa Securities Group and SDGs". https://www.daiwa-grp.jp/english/sdgs/data/pdf/daiwa_sdgs_en_booklet_2020sec.pdf.

contributions toward the enhancement of global health through continuous donations to Doctors Without Borders' Fundraising for Coronavirus Infectious Disease Crisis.[21]

Notably, the Gates Foundation has closely coordinated with these companies, business leaders, international organizations, and nongovernmental organizations. Japan's further contributions to global health are likely what Gates and Kishida discussed in their teleconference, although the exact details of the teleconference have been unknown. For the sake of an early recovery and sustainable growth of the world economy, the Kishida administration must have been encouraged to expand its official development assistance (ODA) for the betterment of global health conditions and formulate Japan's new Global Health Strategy in the COVID-19 pandemic and in preparation for the postpandemic world. In sum, Japanese Business Leaders' Coalition has been committed to the promotion of Japan's global health policy in the world as shown in Table 7.1

## JAPANESE BUSINESS LEADERS
## AND GLOBAL HEALTH ACTION JAPAN 2022

Notably, the Japanese Business Leaders' Coalition for Global Health submitted their policy proposal for global health policy to Prime Minister Kishida on April 22, 2022.[22] In the proposal, Japanese business leaders requested the prime minister to double Japan's global health-related ODA so that Japan could make a greater contribution to the field of ODA and global health.[23] In 2021, Japan was the "fourth-largest OECD DAC donor" to global health, and was "26th among DAC donors" in terms of its prioritization of global health and the size of its overall ODA budget. Japan's global health ODA budget

---

[21] Suntory. 2022. "The Suntory Group's 7 Sustainability Themes". https://www.suntory.com/csr/themes/health/; and see also, Japan News. September 30, 2021. "Suntory Holdings Limited Suntory Group Global Health Management × Sustainability Initiative 'One Suntory Walk'". https://re-how.net/all/1420090/.

[22] Tokyo Shimbun. April 23, 2022. "Kishida Shusho no Ichinichi, April 22 (Prime Minister Kishida's Schedule of April 22)". https://www.tokyo-np.co.jp/article/173402.

[23] PR Times. April 22, 2022. "Japanese Business Leaders' Coalition for Global Health Requested Prime Minister Kishida to Strengthen Japan's Global Health Activities". https://prtimes.jp/main/html/rd/p/000000009.000076537.html.

**Table 7.1**  Japanese business leaders' coalition for global health

| Name of company | Name of leader | Field of contribution to global health |
| --- | --- | --- |
| Shibusawa & Company | Ken Shibusawa | Impact investment for global health |
| Sysmex | Hisashi Ietsugu | Inspection equipment for malaria |
| NEC | Nobuhiro Endo | Child fingerprint identification system |
| Gates Foundation | Mihoko Kashiwakura | Promotion of global health policy |
| SORA Technology | Yosuke Kaneko | Malaria control by AI and drone |
| Toyota Tsusho | Jun Karube | Refrigerated vaccine transport vehicle |
| Fujifilm | Teiichi Goto | Portable X-ray for tuberculosis detection |
| Saraya | Yusuke Saraya | Hand-washing and hand-sanitization |
| Daiwa Securities | Keiko Tashiro | Issuing of vaccine bonds |
| Shionogi | Isao Teshirogi | Development of vaccines and medicines |
| Eisai | Haruo Naito | Medicine to combat lymphatic filariasis |
| Suntory | Takeshi Niinami | Donations to Doctors Without Borders |
| Yamaha Motor | Yoshihiro Hidaka | Clean water system and vaccine transport |

*Note* Created by the author based on this chapter

was nearly doubled during the period from 2019 to 2020, but it was "driven by an increase in bilateral health ODA, which expanded by 48 percent from 2020 levels to support COVID-19 response".[24] Moreover, in comparison with the budget in 2020, the amount of multilateral donation in Japan's global health ODA budget was decreased, while that of the bilateral donation was increased.[25] The Japanese Business Leaders' Coalition for Global Health has consistently argued that the

---

[24] Donor Tracker. July 20, 2023. "Japan / Global Health: ODA Spending". https://donortracker.org/donor_profiles/japan/globalhealth.

[25] Ibid.

Japanese government should reallocate more budget to global health, just as proposed by civil society,[26] as well as in academia.[27]

Moreover, the Japanese Business Leaders' Coalition for Global Health invited Bill Gates to attend Global Health Action Japan as TICAD 8 Official Side Event held in Tokyo on August 19, 2022.[28] On the day, 11 Japanese companies joined the event and made presentations on their activities for global health in front of Bill Gates. Shionogi made a presentation, "Aiming to Protect People Worldwide from the Threat of Infectious Diseases". Saraya introduced their activities in a presentation, "Approach to Global Health: Saraya's Initiative for IPC & NTDs". Sysmex discussed the issue of malaria in its presentation, "Fighting Malaria with Diagnostics". Eisai's presentation was on "Tackling Neglected Tropical Diseases (NTDs)".[29]

Toyota Tsusho made a presentation on "Toyota Tsusho's Last One Mile Initiatives". Sora Technology's presentation was on "SORA Malaria Control", while Yamaha Motor's presentation was on "Yamaha Motor's Role in Global Health". NEC talked about "Technology Innovations for Global Health" and Daiwa Securities made a presentation: "Daiwa had led Vaccine Bond initiative in Japan since 2008". Fujifilm's presentation was on "FUJIFILM Portable X-ray Technology: Vital Equipment in the Worldwide Effort to End Tuberculosis". All these presentations represent the Japanese business leaders' and companies' commitments to global health issues worldwide.[30] On November 14, 2022, the business leaders' coalition requested Foreign Minister Yoshimasa Hayashi to

[26] Japan Center for International Exchange (JCIE). 2021. "Japan's Global Health Diplomacy in the Post-COVID Era: The Paradigm Shift Needed on ODA and Related Policies". Special Commission on Japan's Strategy on Development Assistance for Health. https://www.jcie.org/wp-content/uploads/2021/03/Full-DAH-report-final-web.pdf.

[27] For instance, Nomura, Shuhei, Lisa Yamasaki, Kazuki Shimizu, Cyrus Ghaznavi, and Haruka Sakamoto. 2022. "Japan's Development Assistance for Health: Historical Trends and Prospects for a New Era". *Lancet*. Vol. 22, No. 100403, pp. 1–9. See also de Campos, Rodrigo Pires and Saori Kawai. 2022. "Japan's ODA to Developing Countries in the Health Sector: Overall Trend and Future Prospects". In *Brazil–Japan Cooperation: From Complementarity to Shared Value*. Singapore: Springer, pp. 43–83.

[28] PR Times. August 25, 2022. "Global Health Action Japan 2022". https://prtimes.jp/main/html/rd/p/000000010.000076537.html.

[29] Ibid.

[30] Ibid.

position "global health" as a major pillar of the Development Cooperation Charter, which was later revised in June 2023.[31] By organizing the Global Health Action Japan and requesting the foreign minister to promote global health policy, the business leaders' coalition has placed political influence over the global health policy in Japan.

## Japanese Business Leaders and the Global Health Academy

Notably, the Japanese Business Leaders' Coalition for Global Health has organized study sessions on global health, namely "Global Health Academy". The first Global Health Academy was held on December 5, 2022. NEC, Shionogi, and SORA Technology made presentations on their activities for global health in terms of technology. They also had a talk session on the 100 Days Mission as one of the agenda items of the G7 Hiroshima Summit. As a chair of the Japanese Business Leaders' Coalition for Global Health, Ken Shibusawa explained the purpose of the Global Health Academy, which is a collaboration of the government and companies to contribute to global health by improving access to medicine, etc. NEC stressed the significance of applying cutting-edge AI technology to global health, especially development of universal vaccination.[32]

Specifically, NEC explained their commitment to the 100 Days Mission in collaboration with the Coalition for Epidemic Preparedness Innovations (CEPI). Shionogi made a presentation on their activities for wastewater-based epidemiology in preparation for the next pandemic. SORA Technology talked about how they utilize AI and drone in combatting malaria in developing countries. Finally, the Gates Foundation introduced an idea of establishing so-called Global Health Emergency Corps (GHEC) as a global network of global health experts in preparation for the next pandemic.[33] It can be observed that while NEC and SORA Technology have focused on technological contributions to global

[31] Eisai. November 15, 2022. "Request to Position 'Global Health' as a Major Pillar of the Next Development Cooperation Charter". https://www.eisai.com/sustainability/atm/ntds/activity/030.html.

[32] PR Times. December 9, 2022. "The First Global Health Academy". https://prtimes.jp/main/html/rd/p/000000013.000076537.html.

[33] Ibid.

health, the Gates Foundation has made contributions to the policy and advocacy of global health in Japan and the world.

On March 29, 2023, the second Global Health Academy was held by the Japanese Business Leaders' Coalition for Global Health. In the opening remark, Mihoko Kashiwakura, Head of East Asia Relations of the Gates Foundation,[34] clarified the purpose of the coalition, namely "access to necessary health care for everyone, and a future where everyone in the world is at good health".[35] Notably, Shigeru Omi as the President of the Japan Community Health Care Organization discussed Japan's leadership in infectious diseases and global health. Omi argued that public–private collaboration is important for addressing global health issues from peacetime in preparation for emergency or pandemic.[36] Omi moreover stressed that Japan's contributions to global health in developing countries would eventually benefit Japan itself in many ways.

Following the presentation by Omi, Teiichi Goto as CEO of Fujifilm made a presentation on Fujifilm's contributions to detecting tuberculosis in application of AI and X ray technology. Hisashi Ietsugu as CEO of Sysmex talked about Sysmex's contributions to early detection of malaria by applying its technology. Whereas it takes 15–30 minutes for malaria detection by conventional inspection equipment, it takes only one minute for Sysmex's inspection equipment to detect malaria as well as anemia. Haruo Naito as CEO of Eisai discussed the importance of partnership for controlling NTDs, especially its contribution to combatting lymphatic filariasis through medication.[37]

The third Global Health Academy took place on April 21, 2023. In the third academy, business leaders discussed global health issues in terms of impact investment. Ken Shibusawa touched on the Study Group on Impact Investment for Global Health, and then proposed to discuss the

---

[34] Mihoko Kashiwakura is one of the most active figures who has advocated for the promotion of global health policy in Japan. See, Science Japan. January 6, 2022. "Solving Global Health Issues: Taking on the Challenge through Collaboration with Partners around the World: Interview with Mihoko Kashiwakura, Head of East Asia Relations, Bill & Melinda Gates Foundation". https://sj.jst.go.jp/stories/2022/s0106-01p.html.

[35] PR Times. March 31, 2023. "The Second Global Health Academy". https://prtimes.jp/main/html/rd/p/000000015.000076537.html.

[36] Ibid.

[37] Ibid.

impact investment for global health at the G7 Hiroshima Summit.[38] In this regard, Ken Shibusawa argued that "Japan has long emphasized global health in its overall diplomatic strategy. In addition to that, one of the core components of the Kishida administration's 'new form of capitalism' is 'investing in people', and health is the bedrock of human capital".[39] In a panel discussion, Katsuaki Watanabe as Chairman of Yamaha Motor discussed its commitment to impact investment through the Yamaha clean water system. Likewise, Haruo Naito as CEO of Eisai explained their commitment to impact investment through the improvement of access to medicine.[40]

The fourth Global Health Academy took place on September 6, 2023. The main theme of the academy was global health in terms of health and nutrition of mothers and children. First, Ken Shibusawa delivered an opening speech, introduced the activities of the Business Leaders' Coalition for Global Health, and discussed the issue of growing population in Africa. Second, Monique Vledder as the Head of the Secretariat for the Global Financing Facility for Women, Children and Adolescents (GFF), a multi-stakeholder global partnership housed at the World Bank, made a presentation on the GFF's contribution to the health and nutrition of mothers and children in developing countries. Saraya talked about their activities on safe motherhood project to prevent cervical cancer in Uganda. Shionogi discussed the importance of the "Mother to Mother Shionogi Project" in Ghana. By the project, Shionogi contributed to improving the conditions of pregnant women and safe delivery. NEC introduced medical interview application to a project on health and nutrition of mothers and children in Ghana. This program has been promoted by NEC, Sysmex, and Ajinomoto, in conjunction with the World Food Programme.[41]

---

[38] Kantei. 2023. "The Study Group on Impact Investment for Global Health" (Final Report March 2023 Executive Summary). https://www.kantei.go.jp/jp/singi/kenkou iryou/en/pdf/health_final_report.pdf.

[39] The Government of Japan. June 16, 2023. "Impact Investing in Global Health: Japan's Commitment as a Frontrunner". *KIZUNA*. https://www.japan.go.jp/kizuna/2023/06/impact_investing_in_global_health.html.

[40] PR Times. April 24, 2023. "The Third Global Health Academy". https://prtimes.jp/main/html/rd/p/000000016.000076537.html.

[41] PR Times. September 8, 2023. "The Fourth Global Health Academy". https://prtimes.jp/main/html/rd/p/000000017.000076537.html.

On November 20, 2023, the fifth Global Health Academy took place to discuss the role of Toyota Tsusho and Yamaha Motor in the field of the last one mile activities. Jun Karube as senior executive advisor and former President and CEO of Toyota Tsusho made a presentation on the role of refrigerated vaccine transportation vehicles as well as medical support by drones. Katsuaki Watanabe as Chairman of Yamaha Motor discussed the role of Yamaha's motorbike and medical ship in the field of global health activities. Thus, the business leaders pointed out the collaboration of their commitments to the last one mile activities in land, sea, and air fields. Furthermore, Yoshihide Suga as former prime minister was invited to deliver a speech at the academy. Suga mentioned Japan's contributions to the COVAX Facility as well as the last one mile activities toward the improvement of global health security and attainment of UHC hand in hand with the business leaders in Japan.[42]

## CONCLUSION

As discussed above, the Business Leaders' Coalition for Global Health has played a unique and considerable role in facilitating Japan's global health policy behind the scene. As observed, the Gates Foundation has played an integral role in promoting the business leaders' coalition along with Ken Shibusawa. Japanese companies, such as NEC, Shionogi, Daiwa Securities, Toyota Tsusho, Yamaha Motor, miup, and Sora Technology, have been committed to the improvement of global health in the world. It can be inferred that Japan's global health policy as well as Japan's Global Health Strategy have been influenced by the advocacy of the business leaders' coalition in the post-COVID-19 pandemic period to a certain extent.

On September 20, 2023, Prime Minister Kishida received the Global Goalkeepers Award 2023 "for Japan's leadership focused on health at the G7 Hiroshima Summit and years of immense contribution to global health" awarded by the Gates Foundation.[43] Although Bill Gates has

---

[42] PR Times. November 22, 2023. "The Fifth Global Health Academy". https://prtimes.jp/main/html/rd/p/000000018.000076537.html.

[43] Prime Minister's Office of Japan. September 20, 2023. "Prime Minister Fumio Kishida Receives the 2023 Global Goalkeeper Award". https://japan.kantei.go.jp/101_kishida/diplomatic/202309/20award.html.

been symbolically influential in the activities of the business leaders' coalition, it is true that Japanese companies have made original contributions to the field of global health in developing countries. The 2022 Global Health Action Japan exemplified the advocacy of the business leaders' coalition to inspire the decision-makers in Japan. In addition, attendance of Bill Gates to this symposium represents the influence of the Gates Foundation over the activities of the business leaders' coalition in Japan and the world. Finally, a series of Global Health Academy organized by the business leaders' coalition should be regarded as substantial contributions to the field of global health policy in Japan and the world in the post-pandemic period.

# CHAPTER 8

# Japan and the GFF: For Health and Nutrition of Mothers and Children

**Abstract** In the field of global health, nutrition and health of mothers and children should be regarded as another important issue. The Global Financing Facility for Women, Children and Adolescents (GFF) is a multi-stakeholder global partnership that aims to improve health and nutrition of women, children, and adolescents in developing countries. In essence, the purpose of the GFF is to improve reproductive, maternal, newborn child, adolescent health, and nutrition (RMNCAH-N). Japan's financial contributions to the GFF are of significance to a great deal, since Tokyo supported the inception and development of the GFF. This chapter sheds light on the significance of the World Bank's GFF, and Japan's incremental contributions to the GFF from its inception to the present, especially during the coronavirus pandemic period.

**Keywords** Global Financing Facility for Women · Children and Adolescents (GFF) · Global health · Japan · Reproductive · maternal · newborn child · adolescent health · and nutrition (RMNCAH-N) · Save the Children · World Bank

## INTRODUCTION

In the field of global health, nutrition and health of mothers and children should be regarded as another important issue. The Global Financing Facility for Women, Children and Adolescents (GFF) is a multi-stakeholder global partnership that aims to improve health and nutrition of women, children, and adolescents in developing countries. In essence, the purpose of the GFF is to improve reproductive, maternal, newborn child, adolescent health, and nutrition (RMNCAH-N). The GFF was established in 2015 to contribute to "filling the existing financing gap to implement the United Nations' *Global Strategy for Women's, Children's and Adolescents' Health (2016–2030)*".[1] According to statistical data reported by the GFF in December 2021, undernutrition is related to about 45 percent of child mortality, and anemia leads to some 20 percent of maternal mortality in the world. Moreover, as many as 149 million children under the age of five suffer from growth inhibition due to malnutrition.[2]

So far, it has been observed that the GFF had been developed as an effective financing mechanism for global health, just like Gavi, the Vaccine Alliance and the Global Fund to fight AIDS, Tuberculosis and Malaria (Global Fund).[3] In the middle of the COVID-19 pandemic, mortality rate of women and children doubled the number of those who passed away owing to the coronavirus during the period from March 2020 to June 2021, indicating wider impact of coronavirus pandemic disruption in lower-income nations.[4] Hence, Japan's contributions to the GFF is of significance to a great deal. This chapter sheds light on the significance of the World Bank's GFF, and Japan's incremental contributions to the

[1] Seidelmann, Lisan, Myria Koutsoumpa, Frederik Federspiel, and Mit Philips. 2020. "The Global Financing Facility at Five: Time for a Change?" *Sexual and Reproductive Health Matters*. Vol. 28, No. 2, p. 1.

[2] Japan Center for International Exchange (JCIE). 2021. "The Global Financing Facility for Women, Children and Adolescents (GFF)". https://www.jcie.or.jp/japan/wp/wp-con tent/uploads/2021/12/GFF_Nutrition_full_ENG.pdf.

[3] Salisbury, Nicole A., Gilbert Asiimwe, Peter Waiswa, Ashley Latimer. 2019. "Operationalising the Global Financing Facility (GFF) Model: The Devil Is in the Detail". *BMJ Global Health*. Vol. 4, No. 2, p. 3.

[4] Paton, James. September 29, 2021. "Deaths of Women and Children Show Wider Impact of Pandemic". *Bloomberg*. https://www.bloomberg.com/news/articles/2021-09-29/deaths-of-women-and-children-show-wider-impact-of-pandemic#xj4y7vzkg.

GFF from its inception to the present, especially during the coronavirus pandemic period.[5]

## The Establishment of the GFF: Toward the Achievement of UHC and SDGs

The World Bank contributed to maternal and child health in the field of family planning in the 1970s, child survival and safe motherhood in the 1980s, and reproductive and child health in the 1990s.[6] Given this background, the establishment of the GFF can be regarded as part of the World Bank's endeavors for the improvement of health and nutrition of mothers and children. In 2007, the Health Results Innovation Trust Fund as a multi-donor trust fund was set up by the World Bank.[7] A program, "Every Woman Every Child",[8] was launched in 2010 by former UN Secretary-General Ban Ki-moon to advance health and well-being of women, children, and adolescents, but it lacked sufficient financial support. To address such global health and nutrition issues, the GFF was established by the United Nations and the World Bank at the Financing for Development Conference held on July 13, 2015 in Addis Ababa, Ethiopia.

Where do the funds of the GFF come from? This is a common question in discussing financial contribution to the GFF. The answer to the questions is as follows: "Finances will come, first and foremost, from domestic resources, both public and private".[9] To be more

---

[5] This chapter is based on an earlier version of the draft. See, Akimoto, Daisuke. August 30, 2022. "Japan's Incrementalism in the World Bank's Global Financing Facility". *ISDP Voices*. https://isdp.eu/japans-incrementalism-in-the-world-banks-global-financing-facility/.

[6] Fernandes, Genevie and Devi Sridhar. 2017. "World Bank and the Global Financing Facility". *BMJ*. Vol. 358, p. 3.

[7] Vledder, Monique. 2014. "The Health Results Innovation Trust Fund (HRITF): A Model of Learning to Improve Value for Money in Health Programs". *Healthcare Research Seminar Series*. https://wdi.umich.edu/wp-content/uploads/Announcement-Vledder-other-schools-v22.pdf.

[8] Every Woman Every Child. 2016. "2020 Progress Report on the EWEC Global Strategy". https://www.everywomaneverychild.org.

[9] Jacovella, Diane, Timothy G. Evans, Mariam Claeson, Ruth Kagia, and Ariel Pablos-Mendez. 2016. "Global Financing Facility: Where Will the Funds Come from?" *Lancet*. Vol. 387, No. 10014, p. 122.

specific, the GFF mobilizes additional funding through the combination of grants from a multi-donor trust fund (GFF Trust Fund), financing from the International Development Association (IDA) and the International Bank for Reconstruction and Development (IBRD) and utilizing other domestic and external resources. The GFF is housed at the World Bank and work with several external financiers, such as the US Agency for International Development, the Swedish International Development Cooperation Agency, and the Islamic Development Bank.[10]

The GFF began its support for four "frontrunner" countries (Congo, Ethiopia, Kenya, and Tanzania) and expanded it to other partner countries in Africa, Asia, and Latin America.[11] As a multilateral partnership, the United Nations, the World Bank Group, and the governments of Canada, Norway, and the United States participated in the launch of the GFF. Notably, the Bill & Melinda Gates Foundation (Gates Foundation), Canada, Japan, and the United States announced new financing commitments of 214 million dollars in total. This is an additional commitment to the previous funding of 600 million dollars and 200 million dollars made by Norway and Canada to the GFF Trust Fund.[12]

So far, the GFF has supported 36 low-and middle-income countries, accelerating achievement of universal health coverage (UHC) and the sustainable development goals (SDGs). The GFF's activities have contributed to reducing mortality rates of pregnant mothers, newborn babies, and children under five years old despite the outbreak of the coronavirus pandemic.[13] In December 2021, the Center for Global Development in Washington made three proposals for the GFF: (1) "pursue a deliberate strategy for prioritization of RMNCAH-N services

[10] Saldinger, Adva. July 24, 2018. "A Look at the Global Financing Facility's Goals, Strategies, and Learnings". https://www.devex.com/news/a-look-at-the-global-financing-facility-s-goals-strategies-and-learnings-93165.

[11] Global Financing Facility (GFF). 2022. "Our Response to COVID-19". https://www.globalfinancingfacility.org/where-we-work.

[12] World Bank. July 13, 2015. "Global Financing Facility Launched with Billions Already Mobilized to End Maternal and Child Mortality by 2030". https://www.worldbank.org/en/news/press-release/2015/07/13/global-financing-facility-launched-with-billions-already-mobilized-to-end-maternal-and-child-mortality-by-2030.

[13] Japan Center for International Exchange (JCIE). October 2021. "GFF Monitor". No. 3. https://www.jcie.or.jp/japan/wp/wp-content/uploads/2021/10/6b2a5fd37b47ec2ea21099b0dad69a50-1.pdf.

and products within the realistic budget constraint to advance evidence-based decisions on certain trade-offs, (2) increase transparency and public visibility into GFF-supported activities and funding, especially related to RMNCAH-N product procurement and overall resource tracking, and (3) explore incentives for increased donor co-financing within the framework of World Bank projects as a strategy to pool and channel more resources through government coffers".[14] These recommendations need to be taken into account for the improvement of the GFF activities. In essence, the GFF has made contributions to the attainment of UHC as well as SDGs which are fundamental elements for global health system and human security.

## Japan's Financial Contributions to the GFF

Prior to the establishment of the GFF, Japan made financial contributions to improving health and nutrition situations of developing countries. In 2009, the Japanese government set up the Japan Trust Fund for Scaling Up Nutrition (SUN) Investments, or the Japan Trust Fund,[15] in cooperation with the World Bank.[16] Based on this background, the Japanese government started to make financial contributions to the GFF. The Japan International Cooperation Agency (JICA) also donated 190 million dollars to the GFF, and since then, JICA has been a key partner of the GFF for co-financing, governance, and advocacy activities.[17]

Japan's financial commitments to the GFF are based on its postwar experience of economic recovery during which the World Bank and the international community had financially supported the reconstruction of Japan after World War II. At the UHC Forum held on December 13, 2017 in Tokyo, the Japanese government announced that it would

[14] Keller, Janeen Madar, Rachel Silverman, Julia Kaufman, and Amanda Glassman. 2021. "Prioritizing Public Spending on Health in Lower-Income Countries: The Role of the Global Financing Facility for Women, Children and Adolescents". *CGD Policy Paper*. No. 246, p. 1.

[15] World Bank Group. 2019. "Japan Trust Fund for Scaling Up Nutrition (2017–2018 Annual Report)". https://thedocs.worldbank.org/en/doc/985031597699264502-0090022020/original/JapanTFAnnualReport2019final29July.pdf.

[16] World Bank. May 15, 2018. "Japan Trust Fund for Scaling Up Nutrition". https://www.worldbank.org/en/programs/japan-trust-fund-for-scaling-up-nutrition.

[17] Global Financing Facility (GFF). 2022. "JICA". https://www.globalfinancingfacility.org/japan-international-cooperation-agency.

contribute 50 million dollars to the GFF.[18] In the forum, Katsunobu Kato, Minister of Health, Labour and Welfare, stated: "I firmly believe that these early-stage investments for UHC by the whole government were an important enabling factor in Japan's rapid economic development later on".[19] Likewise, Japan's global health policy and activities of the GFF overlap to a great degree as argued by Shunsuke Mabuchi, a senior advisor of the Gates Foundation, in a report published by the Japan Center for International Exchange (JCIE) in 2021.[20]

At a national political level, Keizo Takemi of the ruling Liberal Democratic Party (LDP) mentioned the significance of the GFF during the Committee on Foreign Affairs and Defense of the Upper House on March 12, 2019.[21] Meanwhile, the nineth meeting of the Diet Caucus on International Maternal and Child Nutrition was held on March 4, 2020, co-organized by Save the Children Japan and Results Japan. Diet members of both ruling parties and opposition parties participated in the meeting and exchanged frank opinions on Japan's policy on maternal and child nutrition in the world.[22] As a coalition government partner of the LDP, Komeito has also been vocal about strengthening the GFF given that "human security" is one of the core pillars of Japan's foreign policy. On December 2, 2021, Kometio officially asked the Japanese

---

[18] Global Financing Facility (GFF). December 14, 2017. "Government of Japan to Invest US$50 Million in Global Financing Facility to Accelerate Progress on Universal Health Coverage". https://www.globalfinancingfacility.org/government-japan-invest-us50-million-global-financing-facility-accelerate-progress-universal-health.

[19] World Bank. December 13, 2017. "World Bank and WHO: Half the World Lacks Access to Essential Health Services, 100 Million Still Pushed into Extreme Poverty Because of Health Expenses". https://www.worldbank.org/en/news/press-release/2017/12/13/world-bank-who-half-world-lacks-access-to-essential-health-services-100-million-still-pushed-into-extreme-poverty-because-of-health-expenses.

[20] Nagatani, Shiori, Tomoko Yoshida, and Tomoko Suzuki. 2021. "Toward Achieving the SDGs: The GFF's Impact and Challenges and Its Significance for Japan". Japan Center for International Exchange (JCIE). https://www.jcie.org/wp-content/uploads/2021/07/GFF-report-2021-EN-070721_1.pdf.

[21] National Diet Library. March 12, 2019. "Proceedings of the 198th Diet Session, Committee on Foreign Affairs and Defense, the House of Councillors". https://kokkai.ndl.go.jp/txt/119813950X00320190312/7.

[22] Results Japan. March 4, 2020. "Minutes of the 9th Diet Caucus on International Maternal and Child Nutrition Progress toward Tokyo Nutrition Summit 2020". http://resultsjp.org/wp/wp-content/uploads/2020/03/Minutes_No9_Diet-Caucus_on_International-Maternal-and-Child-Nutrition_20200304.pdf.

government, especially the Ministry of Finance, to secure sufficient financial support for the GFF prior to the Tokyo Nutrition for Growth Summit 2021.[23] State Minister of Finance Mitsunari Okamoto replied that the government would take the party's request into consideration. On December 7, 2021, an international event entitled, "Investing in Nutrition: Role of Catalytic Financing" was held as an official event of the Tokyo Nutrition for Growth Summit, which was organized by the Japanese government in conjunction with the GFF, the World Bank Group, the Japanese Ministry of Finance, and the JCIE.[24] Clearly, key Japanese lawmakers and policy makers have been aware of the significance of the GFF even in the middle of the coronavirus pandemic.

On June 22, 2023, Save the Children Japan and the JCIE co-organized a study session, "For the sake of All Women and Children's Health: What Is the Role of the Global Financing Facility?" in the First Members' Office Building of the Lower House. Ethiopian Ambassador, Diet members, government officials, non-governmental organizations, youth members who are interested in global health joined the study session.[25] Thus, several Japanese lawmakers and non-governmental organizations (NGOs), such as the JCIE, Save the Children Japan, and Results Japan, have been actively committed to Japan's financial contribution to the GFF overtime including the COVID-19 pandemic period.

## TACKLING INTERNATIONAL AND DOMESTIC POVERTY

One of the major partners of the GFF in civil society is Save the Children that has called on governments, private sectors, and other stakeholders to fund the fight for RMNCAH-N.[26] Hand in hand with Save

---

[23] Komeito. December 3, 2021. "Adequate Financial Contributions to International Organizations". https://www.komei.or.jp/komeinews/p218113/.

[24] Japan Center for International Exchange (JCIE). January 21, 2021. "Investing in Nutrition: Role of Catalytic Financing". https://www.jcie.or.jp/japan/report/activity-report-14687/.

[25] Save the Children Japan. July 3, 2023. "For the Sake of All Women and Children's Health: What Is the Role of the Global Financing Facility?" https://www.savechildren.or.jp/sp/news/index.php?d=4200.

[26] Save the Children. 2018. "The Global Financing Facility: An Opportunity to Get It Right". https://resourcecentre.savethechildren.net/document/global-financing-facility-opportunity-get-it-right.

the Children, the GFF plans to raise 1.2 billion dollars and save additional five million lives in the world by 2025.[27] As shown in Table 8.1, the contribution ratio of the Japanese government among all donors for the GFF is only 3.3 percent in contrast to other top donor countries, such as Norway (29.5 percent), Canada (22 percent), the Netherlands (4.3 percent), and Germany (3.8 percent). Notably, the donation to the GFF by the Gates Foundation amounted to 18.1 percent, which is nearly six times larger than Japan's contribution.[28] This signifies that the international community expects Japan as the fourth largest economy in the world to make further financial contributions to the GFF.[29]

At the same time, the Japanese government would need to pay special attention to domestic poverty among children in Japan. Whereas children in developing countries suffer from absolute poverty, one in seven children in Japan lives in relative poverty as pointed out by the research

**Table 8.1**  Contributions by donors to the GFF and percentage of total

| Donors | Total donation (as of March 2019) | Percentage of total (percent) |
| --- | --- | --- |
| Norway | 448.0 | 29.5 |
| Canada | 334.5 | 22.0 |
| Gates Foundation | 275.0 | 18.1 |
| The UK | 104.1 | 6.9 |
| Buffett Foundation | 75.0 | 4.9 |
| The Netherlands | 66.0 | 4.3 |
| Germany | 58.0 | 3.8 |
| **Japan** | **50.0** | **3.3** |

*Note* Created by the author based on data by the Japan Center for International Exchange

[27] Save the Children. April 22, 2022. "9 Million People Die Every Year from Conditions That Should Be Addressed by Their Health System. What Can Be Done to Change This?" https://www.savethechildren.net/blog/9-million-people-die-every-year-conditions-should-be-addressed-their-health-system-what-can-be.

[28] Japan Center for International Exchange (JCIE). 2021. "The Global Financing Facility for Women, Children and Adolescents (GFF)", p. 6. https://www.jcie.or.jp/japan/wp/wp-content/uploads/2020/09/GFF090920.pdf.

[29] Ibid.

of the Nippon Foundation.[30] According to the Comprehensive Survey of Living Conditions by the Ministry of Health, Labour and Welfare, relative poverty of single-parent households in Japan had been the worst among countries of the Organization of Economic Cooperation and Development (OECD) as reported by *Mainichi Shimbun* on November 27, 2017.[31]

Prime Minister Kishida has argued that his government would facilitate a "virtuous cycle of growth and distribution",[32] as a "new form of capitalism" with a view to "solving social issues the international community faces such as climate change and poverty through public–private partnerships and the promotion of digitization and innovation, while supporting sustainable economic development".[33] Thus, the Japanese government has been in charge of both domestic and international contributions to improving the health and nutrition of women and children. Since the financial contributions to the GFF stem from the tax in Japan, the Japanese government needs to balance the distribution of the budget to the domestic and international contributions.

## Conclusion

As discussed in this chapter, the Japanese government has made continuous financial contributions to the GFF based on its experience of postwar recovery which had been financially supported by the World Bank. Prior to the establishment of the GFF, the Japanese government set up the Japan Trust Fund to improve nutrition and health in developing countries. Minister of Health, Labour and Welfare Katsunobu Kato, Keizo Takemi of the LDP, State Minister of Finance Mitsunari Okamoto showed their strong support for the enhancement of the

[30] Nippon Foundation. 2015. "Addressing Child Poverty". https://www.nippon-fou ndation.or.jp/en/what/projects/ending_child_poverty.

[31] Mainichi Shimbun. November 27, 2017. "Japan Needs Long-term Plan to Tackle Vicious Poverty Cycle". https://mainichi.jp/english/articles/20171127/p2a/00m/0na/016000c.

[32] Prime Minister of Japan and His Cabinet. November 8, 2021. "Outline of Emergency Proposal Toward the Launch of a 'New Form of Capitalism' that Carves Out the Future". https://japan.kantei.go.jp/ongoingtopics/_00001.html.

[33] Prime Minister of Japan and His Cabinet. April 23, 2022. "Speech by Prime Minister KISHIDA Fumio at the 4th Asia–Pacific Water Summit". https://japan.kantei.go.jp/101_kishida/statement/202204/_00017.html.

GFF by increasing Japan's financial contribution to the facility. Likewise, Japanese NGOs, such as the JCIE, Save the Children Japan, and Results Japan, have been continuously active in their advocacy for political and financial support for the GFF.

Hence, it is fair to argue that the Japanese government is expected to make further financial contributions to reducing both global absolute poverty through the support for the GFF and domestic relative poverty in collaboration with domestic programs to end child poverty by NGOs, especially Save the Children Japan,[34] as well as through the Children and Families Agency which was established in April 2023.[35] In sum, Japan's policy toward the GFF and its support for health and nutrition of women, children and adolescents inside the country, have been incremental and meaningful in the coronavirus pandemic period. The Japanese government might as well politically and financially support the GFF in cooperation with the NGOs for the better.

In addition, on April 12, 2023, the Ministry of Finance announced that Japan would make an additional contribution of 10 million dollars to the GFF at the 107th Meeting of the Development Committee, Joint Ministerial Committee of the Boards of Governors of the Bank and the Fund, held in Washington.[36] Furthermore, Japan's contribution to the GFF can eventually contribute to the attainment of UHC in the long run.[37] The Japanese government needs to keep on making further financial contributions to the GFF so that it could save the lives of mothers and children and improve the global health security in the COVID-19 period as well.

[34] Save the Children Japan. 2021. "Save the Children Japan Annual Report 2020". https://www.savechildren.or.jp/news/publications/download/2020_SCJ_AR_English.pdf.

[35] Japan Times. March 24, 2022. "New Agency Aims to Offer Seamless Support for Children in Japan". https://www.japantimes.co.jp/news/2022/03/24/national/japan-children-agency/.

[36] Ministry of Finance Japan. April 12, 2023. "Japan's Statement at the 107th Meeting of the Development Committee (Joint Ministerial Committee of the Boards of Governors of the Bank and the Fund) (Washington, DC—April 12, 2023)". https://www.mof.go.jp/english/policy/international_policy/imf/dc/20230412_2.html.

[37] Hutchison, Hayley. 2023. "The Road to UHC: The GFF's Catalytic Role in Supporting PHC Toward the Achievement of UHC". Japan Center for International Exchange (JCIE). https://www.jcie.org/wp-content/uploads/2023/10/JCIE-GFF-PHC-UHC-Report-final.pdf.

# CHAPTER 9

# Japan, the GHIT Fund, Neglected Tropical Diseases (NTDs)

**Abstract** In the middle of the coronavirus pandemic, the issue of "neglected tropical diseases" (NTDs) tends to be literally neglected, and the term, NTDs, itself is not widely recognized by most people in the world. NTDs are a group of some 20 diseases and conditions mainly prevalent in tropical areas. In recent years, the Japanese government has supported the establishment and development of the "Global Health Innovative Technology Fund" (GHIT Fund) to invest in research and development for combating NTDs. This chapter examines Japan's contributions to controlling and eliminating NTDs by investigating domestic cases in Japan as well as Japan's global health diplomacy in collaboration with the GHIT Fund. This chapter moreover points out the significance of Japan's global health diplomacy at the G7 Hiroshima Summit held on May 19–21, 2023.

**Keywords** Dengue fever · Global Health Innovative Technology Fund (GHIT Fund) · Hansen's disease · Lymphatic filariasis · Neglected tropical diseases (NTDs)

## INTRODUCTION

In the middle of the coronavirus pandemic, the issue of "neglected tropical diseases" (NTDs) tends to be literally neglected, and the term, NTDs, itself is not widely recognized by most people in the world.[1] NTDs are a group of some 20 diseases and conditions mainly prevalent in tropical areas, especially in Africa, Asia, and Latin America. There exists so-called "attention gap" regarding global health agenda,[2] especially "devastating comparison" between NTDs and "big three" infectious diseases, namely HIV/AIDS, tuberculosis, and malaria.[3] Hence, more international attention needs to be paid to NTDs in order to reduce, control, and terminate the diseases. To this end, it is important for the international community to make foreign policy of each country functional for global public health and strengthen global health governance through "global health diplomacy".[4]

The following diseases are categorized as NTDs: Buruli ulcer, chagas disease, cysticercosis, dengue fever, dracunculiasis (Guinea worm disease), echinococcosis, fascioliasis, human African trypanosomiasis (African sleeping sickness), leishmaniasis, Hansen's disease (leprosy), lymphatic filariasis, mycetoma, onchocerciasis, rabies (hydrophobia), schistosomiasis, soil-transmitted helminths (ascaris, hookworm, and whipworm), and trachoma, etc.[5] In terms of Japan's global health diplomacy, Prime Minister Ryutaro Hashimoto contributed to shedding light on the issue of neglected diseases caused by parasites at the event of the G8 Denver

---

[1] World Health Organization (WHO). 2022. "Neglected Tropical Diseases". https://www.who.int/health-topics/neglected-tropical-diseases#tab=tab_1.

[2] Takuma, Kayo. 2020. *Jinrui to Yamai (Humankind and Diseases)*. Tokyo: Chuokoron-Shinsha, p. 207.

[3] Hotez, Peter J. 2020. *Forgotten People Forgotten Diseases: The Neglected Tropical Diseases and Their Impact on Global Health and Development*. Third Edition. Washington D.C.: Wiley, p. 11.

[4] McInnes, Colin and Kelly Lee. 2012. *Global Health and International Relations*. Cambridge: Polity Press, p. 54.

[5] Centers for Disease Control and Prevention (CDC). 2022. "Neglected Tropical Diseases (NTDs)". https://www.cdc.gov/globalhealth/ntd/index.html.

Summit in 1997,[6] and the G8 Birmingham Summit in 1998.[7] The "Global Parasite Control for the 21st Century Initiative" promoted by the Hashimoto government has been known as the "Hashimoto Initiative" in the history of NTDs and global health.[8] Based on the Hashimoto Initiative, the Asian Center of International Parasite Control was established in the Faculty of Tropical Medicine of Mahidol University, Thailand.[9]

In recent years, the Japanese government has supported the establishment of the "Global Health Innovative Technology Fund" (GHIT Fund) to invest in research and development for combating NTDs.[10] NTDs have tended to be overlooked by pharmaceutical companies due to the "lack of market mechanism" as pointed out by Kei Katsuno,[11] and therefore, the Japanese government as well as the GHIT Fund collaboratively facilitate research and development on drugs and medicines to combat NTDs. This chapter examines Japan's contributions to controlling and eliminating NTDs by investigating domestic cases in Japan as well as Japan's global health diplomacy in collaboration with the GHIT Fund. Finally, this chapter points out the significance of Japan's global health diplomacy at the G7 Hiroshima Summit held on May 19–21, 2023.[12]

---

[6] Ministry of Foreign Affairs of Japan. June 22, 1997. "Record on Press Conference by Prime Minister Ryutaro Hashimoto in Denver". https://www.mofa.go.jp/mofaj/gaiko/summit/denver/kaiken.html.

[7] Ministry of Foreign Affairs of Japan. May 15–17, 1998. "G8 Birmingham Summit Communiqué". https://www.mofa.go.jp/mofaj/gaiko/summit/birmin98/commun.html.

[8] Molyneux, David H., Anarfi Asamoa-Bah, Alan Fenwick, Lorenzo Savioli, and Peter Hotez. 2021. "The History of the Neglected Tropical Disease Movement". *Tropical Medicine and Hygiene*. Vol 115, No. 2, pp. 169–175.

[9] Faculty of Tropical Medicine, Mahidol University. 2008. "50th Anniversary of the Faculty of Tropical Medicine, Mahidol University: History". https://www.tm.mahidol.ac.th/50th-anniversary/history.htm.

[10] Abe, Shinzo. September 14, 2013. "Japan's Strategy for Global Health Diplomacy: Why It Matters". *Lancet*. Vol. 382, No. 9896, p. 916.

[11] Katsuno, Kei. 2021. "Japan's Innovation for Global Health: GHIT's Catalytic Role". *Parasitology International*. Vol. 80. https://www.sciencedirect.com/science/article/pii/S1383576920301823?via%3Dihub.

[12] This chapter is based on my earlier research on Japan's policy toward NTDs. See Akimoto, Daisuke. December 2022. "Japan Leads the Way in Global Health Diplomacy: The Case of Neglected Tropical Diseases (NTDs)". *ISDP Issue Brief*, pp. 1–9.

## NTD Cases in Japan: Dengue Fever, Hansen's Disease, and Lymphatic Filariasis

In examining Japan's global health policy toward NTDs, it is important to contextualize how Japan succeeded in controlling and eradicating some NTDs (dengue fever, Hansen's disease, and lymphatic filariasis) domestically. Among NTDs, dengue fever is recognized by most people in Japan. Dengue virus infection is caused by mosquito bites just like other infectious diseases.[13] When a pregnant woman is bitten by an infected mosquito with dengue virus, it could be passed to her fetus during pregnancy or childbirth, causing the death of the fetus and other problems. In the past, epidemics of dengue fever were reported in western part of Japan, especially in cities of Nagasaki, Hiroshima, Kobe, and Osaka, from 1942 to 1945.[14] There was no record of domestic infection of dengue fever inside Japan since then, but it was reported that 162 people of the country were infected by dengue fever in 2014.[15] Although none of them died of the disease, most patients suffered from fevers and headaches. In 2019, there were 461 cases of dengue fever reported in Japan, although the number of cases dramatically dropped to 43 in 2020 and to 8 in 2021, due to the border control for the coronavirus pandemic.[16] Having said that, since infective mosquitoes exist in Japan, further attentions need to be paid to recurrence of outbreak of dengue fever in Japan.

Likewise, Hansen's disease (leprosy) is familiar to Japanese people. Hansen's disease is caused by slow-growing bacteria, mycobacterium leprae, which can affect the nerves, skin, eyes, and noses, and may cause paralysis of hands and feet, and blindness.[17] In Japan, a policy of compulsory isolation of patients of Hansen's disease was implemented by the

[13] Centers for Disease Control and Prevention (CDC). 2022. "Dengue During Pregnancy". https://www.cdc.gov/dengue/transmission/pregnancy.html.

[14] Infectious Disease Surveillance Center. 2000. "Imported Dengue Fever in Japan". *Infectious Agents Surveillance Report*. Vol. 21, No. 6. http://idsc.nih.go.jp/iasr/21/244/tpc244.html.

[15] Uematsu, Yoshika. May 19, 2020. "Dengue Fever Growing Concern in Japan Due to Deadly Mosquito". *Asahi Shimbun*. https://www.asahi.com/ajw/articles/13385845.

[16] Jackson, Alex. June 16, 2022. "Dengue Fever a Growing Threat in Asia". *Japan Times*. https://www.japantimes.co.jp/news/2022/06/16/asia-pacific/science-health-asia-pacific/dengue-fever-asia/.

[17] Centers for Disease Control and Prevention (CDC). 2022. "Hansen's Disease (Leprosy)". https://www.cdc.gov/leprosy/index.html.

Japanese government in 1907.[18] Under the 1953 Leprosy Prevention Law, campaigns to track down patients and forcibly send them to sanatoriums were conducted. The isolation system remained effective until 1996.[19] In May 2001, the Kumamoto District Court ruled that the national government must compensate Hansen's disease patients who had received discriminatory sterilization surgeries. Three days later, Chikara Sakaguchi, as a medical doctor, a lawmaker of Komeito, and Minister of Health, Labour and Welfare, admitted the failure of the government's policy and officially apologized to the patients.[20] Thus, Hansen's disease is thought to be a past disease in Japan, but recent research indicates the rise of non-autochthonous cases due to the result of globalization. Hence, continuous surveillance and public health services for Hansen's disease are necessary even after reaching the state of eradication inside Japan.[21]

Lymphatic filariasis is a parasitic disease caused by microscopic thread-like worms that can live in lymph system of human beings. People get infected by the disease through mosquito bites, and patients suffer from swelling or permanent paralysis of legs.[22] Lymphatic filariasis may not be familiar to most people in Japan, but cases of the disease had been reported in Japan since the Heian period (794–1185).[23] Researchers on the history of pharmacy analyzed that the Meiji Restoration hero Takamori Saigo suffered from lymphatic filariasis, and was not able to

[18] Ishii, Masato. August 17, 2016. "Hansen's Disease in Japan: The Lingering Legacy of Discrimination". *Nippon.com*. https://www.nippon.com/en/features/c02703/?pnum=1.

[19] The Guardian. April 13, 2016. "'Like Entering a Prison': Japan's Leprosy Sufferers Reflect on Decades of Pain". https://www.theguardian.com/world/2016/apr/14/like-entering-a-prison-japans-leprosy-sufferers-sue-government-for-decades-of-pain.

[20] Tadokoro, Ryuko. June 13, 2018. "Former Health Minister Supports Compensation for Forced Sterilization Victims". *Mainichi Shimbun*. https://mainichi.jp/english/articles/20180613/p2a/00m/0na/002000c.

[21] Yotsu, Rie R., Yuji Miyamoto, Shuichi Mori, Manabu Ato, Mariko Sugawara-Mikami, Sayaka Yamaguchi, Masashi Yamazaki, Motoaki Ozaki, and Norihisa Ishii. October 21, 2022. "Hansen's Disease (Leprosy) in Japan, 1947–2020: An Epidemiologic Study during the Declining Phase to Elimination". *International Journal of Infectious Diseases*. https://www.ijidonline.com/article/S1201-9712(22)00565-3/fulltext.

[22] Centers for Disease Control and Prevention (CDC). 2022. "Parasites: Lymphatic Filariasis". https://www.cdc.gov/parasites/lymphaticfilariasis/index.html.

[23] Eisai. 2014. "History of Lymphatic Filariasis Elimination in Japan". https://atm.eisai.co.jp/english/activity/.

ride a horse after being infected by the disease. Lymphatic filariasis was prevalent in Kyushu and Okinawa regions until the 1960s, but owing to the development of medicines, Japan became the first country that succeeded in eliminating the disease by the end of the 1970s.[24] In this context, Kozo Akino as a medical doctor and parliamentary politician of Komeito shed light on Japan's experience of controlling and eradicating lymphatic filariasis in Okinawa during the Committee on Audit of the House of Councillors on May 18, 2011.[25] Akino suggested that the Japanese government should make the best of the Okinawa method to contribute to combatting the disease in the world.[26] In response, the Japanese government pledged that it would attempt to contribute to combatting NTDs, including lymphatic filariasis in developing countries.[27] In short, Japan's experience in controlling and eradicating some NTDs domestically might be contributive to its global health diplomacy for the global control and elimination of NTDs.

## The Global Health Innovative Technology Fund (GHIT Fund)

As shown in domestic cases and experience of Japan, drug discovery and development is critical for controlling and eradicating NTDs,[28] and Japan has been willing to make contributions to reduction and eradication of the diseases. In order to systematically address the reduction of NTDs through effective investment in the development of medicines, vaccines, and diagnostic drugs of infectious diseases in developing countries, the GHIT Fund was established in Tokyo on November 6, 2012.[29] The

[24] Kobayashi, Teruyuki. 2019. "The Control of Lymphatic Filariasis in Japan". *Japanese Journal of History of Pharmacy*. Vol. 54, No. 2, pp. 83–88.

[25] National Diet Library. May 18, 2011. "Proceedings of the 177th Diet Session. The Committee on Audit, the House of Councillors". https://kokkai.ndl.go.jp/txt/117714103X00620110518/195 and https://kokkai.ndl.go.jp/txt/117714103X00620110518/196.

[26] Ibid.

[27] Ibid.

[28] Swinney, David C. and Michael P. Pollastri, eds. 2019. *Neglected Tropical Diseases: Drug Discovery and Development*. Weinheim: Wiley–VCH.

[29] GHIT Fund. 2022. "Global Health Innovative Technology Fund". https://www.ghitfund.org.

headquarters of the GHIT Fund is located in Tokyo, since Japan has one of the largest pharmaceutical industries in the world and possesses a potential for further investment.[30] The Tokyo-based fund was established based on a recognition that "global health" is a central component of Japan's foreign policy.[31] B. T. Slingsby, Executive Director of the GHIT Fund, stated that "If you just look at the number of drugs that are produced by Japanese pharmaceutical companies in general, Japan is number three behind the US and UK. There is an enormous capacity and culture of innovation here in Japan. It's just a matter of how to bring that into global health."[32] The GHIT Fund as a non-profit organization and a "catalyst" of Japan's pharmaceutical sector aims at facilitating the research and development of new medicines to tackle not only three infectious diseases, such as HIV/AIDS, tuberculosis, Malaria, but also NTDs around the world through the public–private partnerships.[33] In other words, the GHIT Fund can be regarded as one of the critical examples of Japan's contributions to the enhancement of global health architecture.

Indeed, the GHIT Fund has been financially supported by funding partners and sponsors, such as the Ministry of Foreign Affairs of Japan, the Ministry of Health, Labour and Welfare of Japan, the United Nations Development Program (UNDP), the Bill & Melinda Gates Foundation (Gates Foundation), and the Wellcome Trust, etc.[34] Japanese pharmaceutical companies, such as Astellas, Chugai, Daiichi Sankyo, Eisai, Shionogi, and Takeda Pharmaceuticals, are also full partners of the fund. Associate partners are Fujifilm, Otsuka, and Sysmex.[35] Overseas companies, such as

---

[30] Nature Medicine. 2013. "Straight Talk with…BT Slingsby". Vol. 19, No. 1553. https://www.nature.com/articles/nm1213-1553.

[31] Slingsby, B. T. and Kiyoshi Kurosawa. 2013. "The Global Health Innovative Technology (GHIT) Fund: Financing Medical Innovations for Neglected Populations". *Lancet Global Health*. Vol. 1, No. 4, pp. 184–185.

[32] Holmes, David. 2013. "The GHIT Fund Shows Its Cards". *Nature Reviews Drug Discovery*. Vol. 12. p. 894.

[33] Otake, Tomoko. December 12, 2017. "Tokyo-Based Fund CEO Leads Public–Private Fight against Diseases around Globe". *Japan Times*. https://www.japantimes.co.jp/news/2017/12/12/national/science-health/tokyo-based-fund-ceo-leads-public-private-fight-diseases-around-globe/.

[34] GHIT Fund. 2022. "Funding Partners and Sponsors". https://www.ghitfund.org/overview/partners.

[35] Ibid.

Johnson & Johnson and Merck, are included as affiliate partners. Sponsors of the GHIT Fund are All Nippon Airways, Yahoo Japan, Salesforce, Zoom, etc.[36] Notably, the financial structure of the fund is composed of the Japanese government (50 percent), pharmaceutical companies (25 percent), and the Gates Foundation and the Wellcome Trust (25 percent). In other words, the GHIT Fund can be regarded as Japan's contribution to pandemic preparedness and enhancement of global health, including measures against NTDs.[37]

Since 2013, the GHIT Fund has invested in 121 cases of research and development of medicines and vaccines with 302 million dollars as of September 27, 2023. In terms of diseases, the GHIT Fund invested 135 million dollars (44.9 percent) in malaria, 30 million dollars (10.0 percent) in tuberculosis, and 136 million dollars (45.2 percent) in NTDs. In the light of intervention by product, the fund invested 200 million dollars (66.2 percent) in drugs, 73 million dollars (24.3 percent) in vaccines, and 28 million dollars (9.5 percent) in diagnostics. As for development stage, 51 million dollars (17.0 percent) was invested in investigated discovery, 160 million dollars (52.8 percent) in preclinical, and 91 million dollars (30.2 percent) in clinical as shown in Fig. 9.1.[38]

The figure shows how the GHIT Fund has been committed to the research and development of medicines and vaccines for the improvement of global health system. In addition, Japanese pharmaceutical companies, such as Astellas, Daiichi Sankyo, Eisai, and Takeda Pharmaceuticals, are included in scope of the 2022 Access to Medicine Index, indicating the global competitiveness and influence over the development of medicines on a global scale.[39] In collaboration with 166 product development partners, the GHIT Fund has contributed to the reduction of major infectious

---

[36] Ibid.

[37] Asian Scientist. September 27, 2019. "Asia's Scientific Trailblazers: Catherine Ohura". https://www.asianscientist.com/2019/09/features/asias-scientific-trailblazers-catherine-ohura-ghit-fund/.

[38] GHIT Fund. 2023. "Investment Overview: Investment to Date Since 2013". https://www.ghitfund.org/investment/overview/jp.

[39] The Access to Medicine Foundation. 2022. *Access to Medicine Index 2022 Methodology*. Amsterdam: The Netherlands, p. 19.

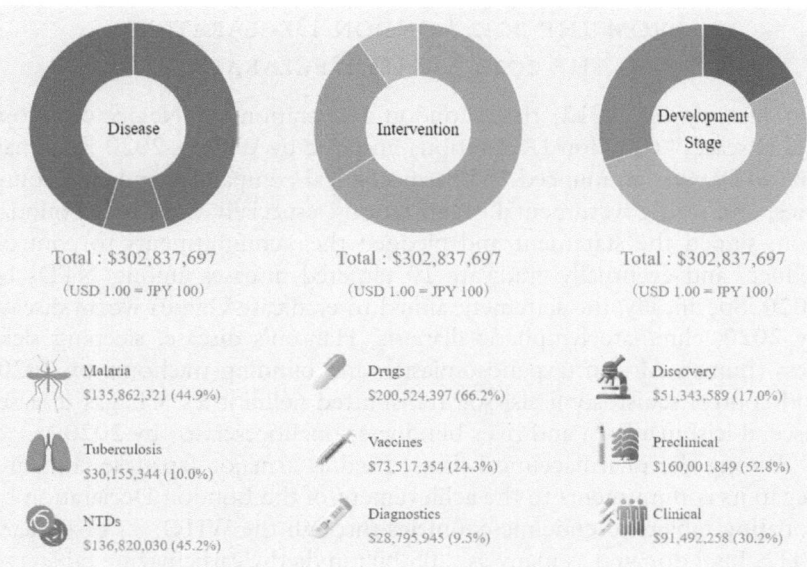

**Fig. 9.1** Breakdown of Investment by the GHIT Fund (*Note* The GHIT Fund uses Japanese yen for investment at 1 US dollar = 100 yen [solely for readers' convenience]. Also, the total percentages in the category of "disease" [malaria, tuberculosis, NTDs] is 101 percent due to rounding)

diseases, such as tuberculosis and malaria, as well as NTDs,[40] representing Japan's contributions to the global health system.

---

[40] GHIT Fund. 2022. "GHIT Fund Annual Report 2021", p. 6. https://www.ghi tfund.org/assets/othermedia/annual_report_2021_eng.pdf.

## From the 2012 London Declaration
## to the 2022 Kigali Declaration

On January 30, 2012, the "London Declaration on Neglected Tropical Diseases" (London Declaration), inspired by WHO's 2020 Roadmap on NTDs, was announced.[41] Pharmaceutical companies, endemic countries, and non-governmental organizations, especially the Gates Foundation, signed the statement and pledged their commitments to control, reduce, and eventually eradicate 10 targeted diseases among NTDs by 2020. Specifically, the statement aimed to eradicate Guinea worm disease by 2020, eliminate lymphatic filariasis, Hansen's disease, sleeping sickness (human African trypanosomiasis), and blinding trachoma by 2020, and control schistosomiasis, soil-transmitted helminthes, Chagas disease, visceral leishmaniasis, and river blindness (onchocerciasis) by 2020.[42]

Among the pharmaceutical firms, Eisai as a major Japanese company began its commitments to the achievement of the London Declaration by donating tablets to endemic countries through the WHO. As of January 2022, Eisai donated as many as 2.05 billion diethylcarbamazine tablets to developing countries suffering from lymphatic filariasis. As a result, the progress of the London Declaration turned out to be measurable and the commitment to reduce NTDs is regarded as a gateway to universal health coverage (UHC).[43] In 2020, 761 million people received medical treatment for NTDs, and at least one NTD has been eliminated in 45 countries so far.[44] From 2012 to 2021, over 17 billion treatments were donated by pharmaceutical industry to defeat NTDs.[45]

On June 24, 2022, the "Kigali Declaration on Neglected Tropical Disease" (Kigali Declaration) was announced during the Global

---

[41] The UK Government. 2012. "London Declaration on Neglected Tropical Diseases". https://assets.publishing.service.gov.uk/government/uploads/system/uploads/attachment_data/file/67443/NTD_20Event_20-_20London_20Declaration_20on_20NTDs.pdf.

[42] Global Health Progress. 2020. "The London Declaration on NTDs". https://globalhealthprogress.org/collaboration/the-london-declaration-on-ntds-2/.

[43] Uniting to Combat NTDs. 2022. "Progress". https://unitingtocombatntds.org/en/neglected-tropical-diseases/progress/; and United to Combat NTDs. 2022. "Reaching a Billion". https://www.infontd.org/resource/reaching-billion-ending-neglected-tropical-diseases-gateway-universal-health-coverage.

[44] Ibid.

[45] Ibid.

Summit on Malaria and Neglected Tropical Diseases (Kigali Summit) held in Kigali of Rwanda.[46] In preparation for this summit, the "Parliamentary League for the Eradication of Neglected Tropical Diseases" formed by Japanese Diet members made policy recommendations for the Kigali Declaration on May 20, 2021. As a top priority in the proposal, the Japanese parliamentary league argued that investment in the GHIT Fund should be expanded.[47] In order to achieve objectives of the Kigali Declaration, the Japanese government needs to collaborate with international organizations, non-governmental organizations, including the Japan Alliance on Global Neglected Tropical Disease (JAGNTD),[48] the Drugs for Neglected Diseases initiative (DNDi),[49] as well as academia, especially the Institute of Tropical Medicine, Nagasaki University.[50] Through the international and multisectoral collaboration, Japan would be able to make more contributions to controlling, reducing, and eliminating the NTDs even in the pandemic period.

## Conclusion

As discussed in this chapter, Japan has made diplomatic and financial contributions to combating NTDs through the Hashimoto Initiative at the 1997 Denver Summit and 1998 Birmingham Summit, the successful control and eradication of its domestic NTDs, the support for the GHIT Fund, and the political advocacy by the Parliamentary League for the Eradication of Neglected Tropical Diseases toward the 2022 Kigali Declaration. As a host country of the 2023 G7 Hiroshima Summit, the Kishida administration made a further contribution to enhancing global health system and expanding its diplomatic and financial contributions to combat NTDs. Indeed, the G7 Hiroshima Leaders' Communique repeatedly

[46] United to Combat NTDs. 2022. "The Kigali Declaration". https://unitingtocom batntds.org/en/the-kigali-declaration/.

[47] The Diet Task Force for Eliminating Neglected Tropical Diseases (NTDs). 2021. "Proposal Commitments by the Government of Japan during the 'Global Summit on Malaria and Neglected Tropical Diseases (Kigali Summit)'". https://jagntd.org/wp-con tent/uploads/2021/06/Policy-recommendations-for-Kigali-Summit-eng.pdf.

[48] Japan Alliance on Global Neglected Tropical Diseases (JAGNTD). 2021. "Japan Alliance on Global Neglected Tropical Disease". https://jagntd.org/.

[49] Drugs for Neglected Diseases initiative (DNDi). 2022. "Drugs for Neglected Diseases initiative". https://dndi.org/#.

[50] Nagasaki University. 2022. "The Institute of Tropical Medicine". https://www.tm. nagasaki-u.ac.jp/nekken/en/.

referred to the term global health and mentioned NTDs as well.[51] Kishida's commitment to global health at the G7 Hiroshima Summit could be recognized as the "Kishida Initiative" to fight against NTDs and to promote the enhancement of global health system in the middle of the COVID-19 pandemic.

Prior to the G7 Ise-Shima Summit, Keizo Takemi, a legislator of the Liberal Democratic Party (LDP), pointed out during the Committee on Health, Labour and Welfare of the House of Councillors on April 21, 2016 that the G7 countries should discuss global health issues including NTDs.[52] During the Ise-Shima G7 Summit held in Mie Prefecture in 2016, the "G7 Ise-Shima Vision for Global Health" was formulated and announced under the leadership of Prime Minister Shinzo Abe.[53] The vision was designed to promote the establishment and enhancement of global health system and pointed out the significance of research and development activities to address NTDs.

Similarly, the Kishida administration successfully included NTDs in the G7 Hiroshima Leaders' Communique in order to control, minimize, and eventually eradicate NTDs, which should not be neglected even during the coronavirus pandemic. This way, the Japanese government took global leadership at the G7 Hiroshima Summit and implemented its global health diplomacy based on the human security policy as its core diplomatic pillar. Likewise, the impact of investment by the GHIT Fund on research and development to combat NTDs could be calculated and visualized in an application of "impact-weighted accounts initiative" (IWAI) promoted by Harvard Business School.[54] In this way, the

---

[51] Ministry of Foreign Affairs of Japan. May 20, 2023. "G7 Hiroshima Leaders' Communiqué". https://www.mofa.go.jp/files/100506907.pdf.

[52] National Diet Library. April 21, 2016. "Proceedings of the 190th Diet Session. Committee on Health, Labour and Welfare, the House of Councillors". https://kokkai.ndl.go.jp/txt/119014260X01520160421/138.

[53] Ministry of Foreign Affairs of Japan. 2016. "G7 Ise-Shima Vision for Global Health". https://www.mofa.go.jp/files/000160273.pdf.

[54] For instance, an impact measurement framework of the "Impact-Weighted Accounts Initiative" (IWAI) of Harvard Business School was applied to an analysis of product impact of pharmaceutical industry. See Rischbieth, Amanda, George Serafeim, and Katie Trinh. 2021. "Accounting for Product Impact in the Pharmaceuticals Industry". *Harvard Business School Working Paper*. 21–139, pp. 1–20. https://www.hbs.edu/impact-weighted-accounts/Documents/Accounting%20for%20Product%20Impact%20in%20the%20Pharmaceuticals%20Industry.pdf?csf=1&web=1&e=8Pells.

future Japanese government and private sectors can make further financial contributions to the GHIT Fund to combat NTDs and to the enhancement of the changing "global health architecture" in the post-COVID-19 era.[55]

[55] "Global health architecture" was considered one of the core themes of the 2023 G7 Hiroshima Summit. See, Japan Center for International Exchange (JCIE). 2022. "Hiroshima G7 Global Health Task Force". https://www.jcie.org/programs/global-health-and-human-security/executive-committee-on-global-health-and-human-security/2023-g7-ghtaskforce/.

# CHAPTER 10

# Japan's Global Health Strategy and the 2023 G7 Hiroshima Summit

**Abstract** On May 19–21, 2023, the Japanese government hosted the G7 Hiroshima Summit. Alongside several global issues, attentions were paid to "global health" at the summit in the wake of the coronavirus pandemic. How has Japan been committed to the G7/G8 summits as a host nation for the sake of global health? This chapter intends to provide an overview of Japan's Global Health Strategy announced by the Kishida administration in May 2022, which became a foundation for Japan's human security diplomacy toward the G7 Hiroshima Summit. Next, it examines the significance of Japan's summit diplomacy for global health by contextualizing Japan's summit diplomacy from the 2000 G8 Kyushu-Okinawa Summit to the 2023 G7 Hiroshima Summit. Finally, this chapter considers policy implications of the G7 Hiroshima Summit for Japan's global health policy during the COVID-19 period.

**Keywords** Coronavirus (COVID-19) · Global Health Strategy · G7 Hiroshima Summit · Japan · Kishida · Summit diplomacy

# INTRODUCTION

On May 19–21, 2023, the Japanese government hosted the G7 Hiroshima Summit. It was assumed that Prime Minister Fumio Kishida planned to express a strong diplomatic message for peace and nuclear disarmament by announcing a so-called "Hiroshima Action Plan" at the summit.[1] Global issues, such as world economy, food deficiency, and energy problem, were on the summit agenda. At the same time, attentions were paid to "global health" at the summit in the wake of the coronavirus pandemic. During TICAD 8 held in Tunisia on August 27–28, 2022, Kishida pledged to donate as much as 1.08 billion dollars to the Global Fund to Fight AIDS, Tuberculosis and Malaria,[2] representing its commitment to global health through the Africa diplomacy.

Notably, a number of policy proposals and academic papers on the G7 Hiroshima Summit from the perspective of global health have been published.[3] The Health and Global Policy Institute (HGPI) submitted a policy proposal to Prime Minister Kishida toward the G7 Hiroshima Summit. The HGPI's proposal stressed the importance of planetary health including measures against climate change.[4] Hiroshima G7 Global Health Task Force in cooperation with the Japan Center for International Exchange (JCIE) published an article with policy recommendations, entitled "Promoting Global Solidarity to Advance Health System Resilience: Recommendations for the G7 Meetings in Japan".[5] Hiroshima G7 Global Health Task Force also published an article in *Lancet* as a policy proposal

---

[1] Japan News. August 28, 2022. "Nuclear Disarmament on Kishida's Mind for Hiroshima G7 Summit Next Year". https://japannews.yomiuri.co.jp/politics/politics-gov ernment/20220828-54608/.

[2] Japan Times. August 29, 2022. "Kishida Shows Leadership at TICAD on Global Health and Security". https://www.japantimes.co.jp/opinion/2022/08/29/com mentary/japan-commentary/japan-ticad-pledge/.

[3] As for one of the proposals and earlier version of this chapter, see Akimoto, Daisuke. September 21, 2022. "Japan's Global Health Strategy: A Diplomatic Foresight on the G7 Hiroshima Summit". *ISDP Voices*. https://isdp.eu/japans-global-health-strategy-a-diplom atic-foresight-on-the-g7-hiroshima-summit/.

[4] Health and Global Policy Institute (HGPI). April 20, 2022. "[Policy Recommenda-tions] Recommendations for the G7 Hiroshima Summit by the C7 Global Health Working Group". https://hgpi.org/en/research/ph-20230420.html.

[5] Hiroshima G7 Global Health Task Force, Executive Committee on Global Health and Human Security. 2023. "Promoting Global Solidarity to Advance Health System

toward the G7 Hiroshima Summit.[6] Moreover, Yudai Kaneda, Kenzo Takahashi, Akihiko Ozaki, and Tetsuya Tanimoto suggested that the G7 countries are responsible for making an international vaccine distribution system more equal given the fact that "vaccine supply faces severe disparities" despite the efforts by the COVID-19 Vaccines Global Access (COVAX) Facility.[7] Obviously, researchers on Japan's global health policy focused on the significance of the G7 Hiroshima Summit since the summit was held during the coronavirus pandemic period.

What is the nature of Japan's Global Health Strategy? How has Japan been committed to the G7/G8 summits as a host nation for the sake of global health? This chapter intends to provide an overview of Japan's Global Health Strategy announced by the Kishida administration in May 2022, which was a foundation for Japan's human security diplomacy toward the G7 Hiroshima Summit. Next, it examines implications of Japan's summit diplomacy for global health by contextualizing Japan's summit diplomacy from the 2000 G8 Kyushu-Okinawa Summit to the 2023 G7 Hiroshima Summit. Finally, this chapter considers policy implications of the G7 Hiroshima Summit for Japan's global health policy during the COVID-19 period.

## JAPAN'S GLOBAL HEALTH STRATEGY BY THE KISHIDA ADMINISTRATION

On May 24, 2022, the Kishida administration set forth its new "Global Health Strategy" as announced by the Office of Healthcare Policy of the Cabinet Secretariat.[8] The document outline in English stresses the significance of "human security", stating that "Health is an essential basis

Resilience: Recommendations for the G7 Meetings in Japan". Japan Center for International Exchange (JCIE). https://www.jcie.org/wp-content/uploads/2023/04/Hiroshima-G7-Global-Health-Task-Force-Recommendations.pdf.

[6] Hiroshima G7 Global Health Task Force. 2022. "Promote Global Solidarity to Advance Health-System Resilience: Proposals for the G7 Meetings in Japan". *Lancet*. Vol. 401, No. 10385, pp. 1319–1321.

[7] Kaneda, Yudai, Kenzo Takahashi, Akihiko Ozaki, and Tetsuya Tanimoto. 2023. "Global Vaccine Equity: The G7's Commitment and Challenge". *GHM Open*. Letter, pp. 1–2.

[8] Prime Minister of Japan and His Cabinet. May 24, 2022. "Global Health Strategy of Japan". https://www.kantei.go.jp/jp/singi/kenkouiryou/en/pdf/final_GHS.pdf.

for development and economic policies, and is fundamental to human security, of which Japan has been a strong proponent".[9] The strategy has two policy goals: (1) to contribute to developing resilient "global health architecture" for international health security and strengthening "prevention, preparedness, and response" (PPR) for public health crises, and (2) to accelerate the efforts to achieve more "resilient, equitable, and sustainable" universal health coverage (UHC).[10] Thus, it is clear that Japan's Global Health Strategy has been based on its human security policy toward the attainment of global health security, UHC, PPR in the post-pandemic world.

The strategy intends to strengthen the global health architecture and to achieve UHC by following these guiding principles: (1) health systems' strengthening at the country level, (2) resilience, (3) equity, and (4) sustainability. To attain the policy goals based on the guiding principles, a "cross-sectoral approach" is proposed with actions in the fields of education, water and sanitation, nutrition, population and development, gender equality, and the empowerment of women.[11] Specifically, actions to be taken in the strategy include: (1) "global health architecture for UHC, (2) partnership with multilateral organizations including the establishment of a WHO's UHC Center in Japan, (3) bilateral cooperation through official development assistance (ODA), such as grant aid, loan, and technical cooperation, (4) multi-stakeholder engagement with civil society organizations, (5) response to various challenges in global health, and (6) cross-sectoral approach".[12]

Evidently, Japan's Global Health Strategy has profound implications for the agenda setting of the G7 Hiroshima Summit in the COVID-19 pandemic. Based on the strategy, Prime Minister Kishida published an article, "Human Security and Universal Health Coverage: Japan's Vision for the G7 Hiroshima Summit" in *Lancet* on January 28, 2023.[13] In the article, Kishida emphasized the significance of human security and

---

[9] Prime Minister of Japan and His Cabinet. 2022. "Global Health Strategy Outline". https://www.kantei.go.jp/jp/singi/kenkouiryou/en/pdf/final_GHS_outline.pdf.

[10] Ibid.

[11] Ibid.

[12] Ibid.

[13] Kishida, Fumio. January 28, 2023. "Human Security and Universal Health Coverage: Japan's Vision for the G7 Hiroshima Summit". *Lancet*. Vol. 401, No. 10373, pp. 246–247.

UHC toward the post-COVID-19 era.[14] In order to figure out how Japan's Global Health Strategy has been shaped overtime, it is necessary to contextualize its summit diplomacy from the G8 Kyushu-Okinawa Summit to the G7 Hiroshima Summit.

## GLOBAL HEALTH AGENDA IN TOKYO'S SUMMIT DIPLOMACY

Japan's global health policy has profound implications for Tokyo's summit diplomacy, through which the Japanese government has made diplomatic contributions to the development of "global health architecture". First, Japan made a diplomatic contribution by proposing an international partnership to fight AIDS, tuberculosis, and malaria at the event of the G8 Kyushu-Okinawa Summit held on July 21–23, 2000.[15] In the Communique Okinawa 2000, G8 countries agreed on implementing an ambitious plan to address HIV/AIDS, tuberculosis, and malaria.[16] Significantly, the establishment of the Global Fund to Fight AIDS, Tuberculosis and Malaria (Global Fund) was based on a proposal by Prime Minister Yoshiro Mori at the Discussion Group on the Kyushu-Okinawa Summit held on June 5, 2000.[17]

Second, prior to the G8 Hokkaido-Toyako Summit held on July 7–9, 2008,[18] Prime Minister Yasuo Fukuda made these opening remarks: "From Okinawa to Toyako: Dealing with Communicable Diseases as Global Human Security Threats" on May 23, 2008.[19] Fukuda's speech

---

[14] Ibid, p. 247.

[15] Ministry of Foreign Affairs of Japan. July 21–23, 2000. "Kyushu-Okinawa Summit". https://www.mofa.go.jp/policy/economy/summit/2000/index.html.

[16] Ministry of Foreign Affairs of Japan. July 23, 2000. "G8 Communique Okinawa 2000". https://www.mofa.go.jp/policy/economy/summit/2000/documents/communique.html.

[17] The Global Fund. 2022. "The Global Fund to Fight AIDS, Tuberculosis and Malaria". https://www.theglobalfund.org/en/.

[18] Ministry of Foreign Affairs of Japan. 2008. "G8 Hokkaido-Toyako Summit". https://www.mofa.go.jp/policy/economy/summit/2008/index.html.

[19] Ministry of Foreign Affairs of Japan. May 23, 2008. "Opening Remarks by H.E. Mr. Yasuo Fukuda, Prime Minister of Japan on the Occasion of 'From Okinawa to Toyako: Dealing with Communicable Diseases as Global Human Security Threats'". https://www.mofa.go.jp/policy/health_c/remark0805.html.

highlighted that global health issues, especially communicable diseases, should be regarded as human security threats. As one of the outcome documents of the summit, the "Toyako Framework Action for Global Health" was formulated and published by the Ministry of Foreign Affairs of Japan.[20] The framework confirmed the necessity of a comprehensive approach toward "health-related" millennium development goals (MDGs) as well as a cross-sectoral approach against infectious diseases, such as HIV/AIDS, tuberculosis, malaria, polio, and neglected tropical diseases (NTDs). In addition, the "Report of the G8 Health Experts Group" containing policy recommendations and data on global health issues was submitted to the G8 countries in the middle of the summit.[21]

Third, the Japanese government highlighted the importance of global health at the G7 Ise-Shima Summit held on May 26–27, 2016.[22] Outcome documents of the summit were on quality infrastructure investment, global health, capacity building of women and girls, cybersecurity, anti-corruption, and anti-terrorism. Notably, the G7 countries announced the "G7 Ise-Shima Vision for Global Health" with concrete action plans,[23] such as the reinforcement of the global health architecture, attainment of UHC, antimicrobial resistance (AMR), and research and development (R&D) for innovative medicine initiative. Prior to the G7 Ise-Shima Summit, an academic paper with policy proposals for the summit was submitted by the "Japan Global Health Working Group", and was published by *Lancet* on May 21, 2016.[24]

With a view to protecting human security, the research proposed three areas of global health: (1) "restructuring of the global health architecture so that it enables preparedness and responses to health emergencies, (2) development of platforms to share best practices and harness shared

---

[20] Ministry of Foreign Affairs of Japan. July 2008. "Toyako Framework Action for Global Health". https://www.mofa.go.jp/policy/economy/summit/2008/doc/pdf/200 80728_02.pdf.

[21] Ministry of Foreign Affairs of Japan. July 8, 2008. "Toyako Framework for Action on Global Health: Report of the G8 Health Experts Group". https://www.mofa.go.jp/policy/economy/summit/2008/doc/pdf/0708_09_en.pdf.

[22] Ministry of Foreign Affairs of Japan. May 27, 2016. "G7 Ise-Shima Summit". https://www.mofa.go.jp/ecm/ec/page4e_000457.html.

[23] Ministry of Foreign Affairs of Japan. 2016. "G7 Ise-Shima Vision for Global Health". https://www.mofa.go.jp/files/000160273.pdf.

[24] Japan Global Health Working Group. 2016. "Protecting Human Security: Proposals for the G7 Ise-Shima Summit in Japan". *Lancet*. Vol. 387, No. 10033, pp. 2155–2162.

learning about the resilience and sustainability of health systems, and (3) strengthening of coordination and financing for research and development and system innovations for global health security".[25] Notably, the Coalition for Epidemic Preparedness Innovations (CEPI) was established as one of the outcomes of the G7 Ise-Shima Summit, which could be regarded as another case of Japan's contribution to global health architecture alongside with the establishment of the Global Fund.

Clearly, Japan's previous diplomatic efforts for global health at G7/G8 summits were consistent and evolutionary even in the pre-COVID-19 period. As already mentioned at the outset, the G7 Hiroshima Summit was hosted by the Kishida administration and global health issues were discussed.[26] In preparation for the summit, the JCIE set up the "Hiroshima G7 Global Health Task Force" under the Executive Committee on Global Health and Human Security chaired by Keizo Takemi, a Diet Member of the House of Councillors, and JCIE President Akio Okawara to make policy recommendations regarding the G7 agenda.[27] Moreover, the JCIE conducted "Hiroshima G7 Global Health Follow-Up Initiative Kick-off Event: Reflections on the 2023 G7" on June 27, 2023. The title of the follow-up event was "Global Health Multistakeholder Dialogue: From Hiroshima to Puglia", and the JCIE organized the event in cooperation with the Bill & Melinda Gates Foundation (Gates Foundation), CEPI, the International Pandemic Preparedness Secretariat, and the Wellcome Trust.[28] The participants of the event discussed how to realize the G7 commitments, especially in the field of PPR.[29] Then, what were outcomes of the G7 Hiroshima Summit in relations with global health?

---

[25] Ibid.

[26] Prime Minister's Office of Japan. 2023. "G7 Hiroshima Summit". https://www.kantei.go.jp/g7hiroshima_summit2023/index.html.

[27] Japan Center for International Exchange (JCIE). 2022–2023. "Hiroshima G7 Global Health Task Force". https://www.jcie.org/programs/global-health-and-human-security/executive-committee-on-global-health-and-human-security/2023-g7-ghtaskforce/.

[28] Japan Center for International Exchange (JCIE). June 27, 2023. "Hiroshima G7 Global Health Follow-Up Initiative Kick-off Event: Reflections on the 2023 G7". https://www.jcie.org/programs/global-health-and-human-security/executive-committee-on-global-health-and-human-security/2023-g7-ghtaskforce/hiroshima-g7-follow-up-initiative-kickoff/.

[29] Ibid.

## GLOBAL HEALTH AGENDA
## IN THE G7 HIROSHIMA SUMMIT

Prior to the G7 Hiroshima Summit, the G7 Health Ministers' Meeting was held in Nagasaki on May 13–14, 2023.[30] First, the G7 health ministers agreed to "develop and strengthen global health architecture for public health emergencies" in terms of governance, coordination framework between health and finance, etc.[31] Second, they agreed to "contribute to achieving more resilient, equitable and sustainable universal health coverage through strengthening health systems"[32] and to "promote health innovation to address various health challenges".[33] In addition, the G7 health ministers agreed on "G7 Global Plan for UHC Action Agenda" and decided to promote "action-oriented global health agenda.[34] It was meaningful to hold the G7 Health Ministers' Meeting in another atomic-bombed city in Japan given the humanitarian implications of the use of nuclear weapons for global health and human beings.

The G7 Hiroshima Leaders' Communique repeatedly mentioned global health, representing that global health was one of the critical issues and agenda items in the post-pandemic summit.[35] The G7 countries expressed their determination to work together in order to "invest in global health through vaccine manufacturing capacity worldwide, the Pandemic Fund, the future international agreement for pandemic prevention, preparedness and response, and efforts to achieve universal health coverage".[36] Regarding the financial contribution to the Pandemic Fund, Japan as the fifth largest donor has made 70 million dollars of donation to

[30] Ministry of Health, Labour and Welfare of Japan. May 13–14, 2023. "G7 Health Ministers' Meeting in Nagasaki". https://www.mhlw.go.jp/stf/seisakunitsuite/bunya/hokabunya/kokusai/g8/g7health2023_en.html.

[31] Ministry of Health, Labour and Welfare of Japan. May 13–14, 2023. "G7 Nagasaki Health Ministers' Communiqué". https://www.mhlw.go.jp/content/10500000/001098603.pdf.

[32] Ibid., pp. 10–14.

[33] Ibid., pp. 15–19.

[34] Ministry of Health, Labour and Welfare of Japan. May 13–14, 2023. "G7 Global Plan for UHC Action Agenda". https://www.mhlw.go.jp/content/10500000/001098604.pdf.

[35] Ministry of Foreign Affairs of Japan. May 20, 2023. "G7 Hiroshima Leaders' Communiqué". https://www.mofa.go.jp/files/100506907.pdf.

[36] Ibid., p. 2.

the fund as of November 4, 2023.[37] The Communique also confirmed the significance of the G7's commitment to develop the global health architecture and global health emergency corps, and to attain UHC and sustainable development goals (SDGs).[38]

Moreover, the Communique agreed to tackle "communicable diseases including HIV/AIDS, tuberculosis, hepatitis, malaria, polio, measles, cholera, and neglected tropical diseases (NTDs), AMR, non-communicable diseases (NCDs) including mental health conditions, realizing comprehensive sexual and reproductive health and rights for all, and promoting routine immunization, healthy ageing, water, sanitation and hygiene".[39] Likewise, it reconfirmed the significance of the G7's contributions to the Global Fund, the Global Polio Eradication Initiative (GPEI), Gavi, the Vaccine Alliance, Global Health Innovative Technology (GHIT) Fund, Coalition for Epidemic Preparedness Innovations (CEPI).[40] The G7 members furthermore agreed on "G7 Hiroshima Vision for Equitable Access to Medical Countermeasure" to improve "equitable access to medical countermeasures for health emergencies" with a view to strengthening global health architecture.[41]

As shown in Table 10.1, Japan as a host country has made diplomatic contributions to the development of global health agenda in G7/G8 summits. In the G8 Kyushu-Okinawa Summit, Japan made a diplomatic contribution to the establishment of the Global Fund. In the G8 Hokkaido-Toyako Summit, Japan's diplomatic leadership led to the "Toyako Framework Action for Global Health". The G7 Ise-Shima Summit became a foundation for the establishment of CEPI. In preparation for the G7 Hiroshima Summit, the Kishida administration formulated Japan's "Global Health Strategy" and has promoted Japan's global health policy in the midst of the coronavirus pandemic. Accordingly, it can be argued that the G7/G8 summits provided opportunities

---

[37] World Bank. November 4, 2023. "The Pandemic Fund". https://fiftrustee.worldb ank.org/en/about/unit/dfi/fiftrustee/fund-detail/pppr.

[38] Ibid., pp. 22–23.

[39] Ibid., p. 24.

[40] Ibid., p. 24–25.

[41] Ministry of Foreign Affairs of Japan. 2022. "G7 Hiroshima Vision for Equitable Access to Medical Countermeasure". https://www.mofa.go.jp/files/100506811.pdf.

**Table 10.1**   Tokyo's G7/G8 summit diplomacy for global health

| Year | G7/G8 summit in Japan | Policy outcomes related to global health |
| --- | --- | --- |
| 2000 | Kyushu-Okinawa | Establishment of the Global Fund (2002) |
| 2008 | Hokkaido-Toyako | "Toyako Framework Action for Global Health" |
| 2016 | Ise-Shima | Establishment of CEPI (2017) |
| 2023 | Hiroshima | Japan's "Global Health Strategy" (2022) |

*Note* Created by the author based on this chapter

with Japan to take diplomatic leadership for enhancing the global health architecture in the pre-and post-COVID-19 pandemic period.

## Conclusion

This chapter has examined Japan's Global Health Strategy, the development of Tokyo's summit diplomacy toward the G7/G8 summits in Japan, and outcomes of the G7 Hiroshima Summit with regards to global health security. Based on "human security" as Japan's diplomatic pillar, the Kishida government made diplomatic contributions toward the G7 Hiroshima Summit in the two main agenda items: (1) promotion of nuclear nonproliferation and disarmament, and (2) global health architecture. Hiroshima is an electoral district of Prime Minister Kishida, and he was enthusiastic about making abolition of nuclear weapons a core summit agenda item, stating: "I would like to make the summit a place for the leaders to show a strong commitment from Hiroshima to never repeating the horrors of nuclear weapons and opposing military aggressions".[42] Given the influence over human body and global health, issues on abolition of nuclear weapons are overlapped with the purpose of global health security.

It is understandable for Kishida to prioritize the issue of nuclear weapons abolition in the summit, and the Japanese government also made global health one of the summit agenda items due to the influence of the COVID-19 pandemic. Theoretically, these two issues are core themes of the human security agenda. According to a final report by the Commission on Human Security co-chaired by Sadako Ogata and Amartya Sen,

[42] Japan Times. June 28, 2022. "Japan to Host G7 Summit in Hiroshima Next May". https://www.japantimes.co.jp/news/2022/06/28/national/g7-hiroshima-summit/.

the definition of human security is "to protect the vital core of all human lives in ways that enhance human freedom and human fulfillment".[43] More specifically, human security is composed of three types of freedom: (1) freedom from fear, (2) freedom from want, and (3) freedom to live in dignity.[44] Whereas abolition of nuclear weapons can be categorized as freedom from fear, enhancement of the global health system is surely categorized as freedom from want, although there may be some overlapping aspects in these two categories.

Prime Minister Kishida's Global Health Strategy is therefore consistent with Japan's human security diplomacy through the presidency of G7/G8 summits. At the G7 Hiroshima Summit, Prime Minister Kishida could have negotiated with other G7 countries about a possibility of adopting a so-called "no first use" of nuclear weapons as part of the Hiroshima Action Plan.[45] The declaration of the non-first use of nuclear weapons has been increasingly regarded as important since the outbreak of the Russia-Ukraine War, and Kishida should have pursued the declaration at the summit as it has profound implications for global health security as well. At any rate, the Kishida administration made a significant diplomatic contribution to emphasizing the significance of global health as one of the G7 summit agenda items based on Japan's Global Health Strategy in the middle of the pandemic period and in preparation for the next pandemic.

[43] United Nations. 2003. "Human Security Now: Protecting and Empowering People". https://digitallibrary.un.org/record/503749?ln=en.

[44] Japan International Cooperation Agency (JICA). January 2021. "Special Report Revisiting Human Security in Today's Context Security and Dignity for All". https://www.jica.go.jp/english/publications/j-world/2101_03.html.

[45] Asahi Shimbun. August 8, 2022. "U.N. Chief Urges Nuke Powers to Abide by No-First-Use Pledge". https://www.asahi.com/ajw/articles/14690104.

# CHAPTER 11

# Japan and CEPI: In Preparation for the Next Pandemic

**Abstract** Prior to the occurrence of the coronavirus (COVID-19) pandemic, the "Coalition for Epidemic Preparedness Innovations" (CEPI) was launched at the annual meeting of the World Economic Forum at Davos in January 2017. Japan, Norway, Germany, the United Kingdom, Canada, Belgium, the Bill & Melinda Gates Foundation (Gates Foundation), and the Wellcome Trust have financially supported the activities of CEPI with a view to facilitating the development of vaccines and equal distribution to developing countries that are under the risk of new infectious diseases. This chapter sheds light on the role of CEPI in preparation for and prevention of the next pandemic in the post-COVID-19 world. To this end, it contextualizes Japan's contributions to the establishment of CEPI, analyzes domestic factor that has facilitated Japan's policy on CEPI, and pays attention to so-called 100 days mission of CEPI in preparation for future pandemics.

**Keywords** Coalition for Epidemic Preparedness Innovations (CEPI) · Coronavirus (COVID-19) · Komeito · Next pandemic · 100 days mission

D. Akimoto, *Japan and Global Health*, https://doi.org/10.1007/978-981-97-0972-4_11

## Introduction

Prior to the occurrence of the coronavirus (COVID-19) pandemic, the Coalition for Epidemic Preparedness Innovations (CEPI) was launched at the annual meeting of the World Economic Forum at Davos in January 2017.[1] CEPI was "formed in the aftermath of the 2014–2015 Ebola outbreak in west Africa to support the development of vaccines that could improve the world's preparedness against outbreaks of epidemic infectious diseases".[2] In essence, CEPI was initiated as a "billion-dollar project" in order to develop and prepare necessary vaccines prior to the outbreak of endemics or pandemics. Japan, Norway, Germany, the United Kingdom, Canada, Belgium, the Bill & Melinda Gates Foundation (Gates Foundation), and the Wellcome Trust have financially supported the activities of CEPI with a view to facilitating the development of vaccines and equal distribution to developing countries that are under the risk of new infectious diseases.[3]

In essence, CEPI is an innovative global partnership between public, private, philanthropic, and civil organizations, to accelerate the development of vaccines against epidemic and pandemic threats. Specifically, CEPI has contributed to developing vaccines against infectious diseases, such as Ebola virus disease, Lassa virus, Middle East Respiratory Syndrome coronavirus, Nipah virus, Rift Valley Fever virus, and Chikungunya virus.[4] The Japanese government has politically and economically supported CEPI, and Komeito as a ruling party has played an integral role in promoting financial contributions to CEPI. This chapter sheds light on the role of CEPI in preparation for and prevention of the next pandemic in the post-COVID-19 world. To this end, it contextualizes Japan's contributions to the establishment of CEPI, analyzes domestic

---

[1] CEPI. 2023. "CEPI: Preparing for Future Pandemics". https://cepi.net.

[2] Gouglas, Dimitrios, Mario Christodoulou, Stanley A. Plotkin, and Richard Hatchett. 2019. "CEPI: Driving Progress Toward Epidemic Preparedness and Response". *Epidemiologic Reviews*. Vol. 41, No. 1, p. 28, pp. 28–33.

[3] Butler, Declan. 2017. "Billion-Dollar Project Aims to Prep Vaccines before Epidemics Hit". *Nature*. Vol. 541, No. 7638, pp. 444–445.

[4] CEPI. 2023. "CEPI: Priority Diseases". https://cepi.net/research_dev/priority-diseases/.

factor that has facilitated Japan's policy on CEPI, and pays attention to so-called 100 days mission of CEPI in preparation for future pandemics.[5]

## JAPAN'S CONTRIBUTIONS TO THE ESTABLISHMENT OF CEPI

CEPI was founded based on an outcome document of the G7 Ise-Shima Summit in 2016 hosted by Prime Minister Shinzo Abe. The Abe government was dedicated to the hosting of the summit, and in the outcome document called the G7 Ise-Shima Vision for Global Health, the G7 countries proposed to "explore the feasibility of partnerships such as the Vaccine Innovation for Pandemic Preparedness Partnership to conduct a coordinated vaccine research and development".[6] In this context, the Japanese government supported the establishment of CEPI in the annual meeting of the World Economic Forum in 2017, and has consistently made political and financial contributions to CEPI.

At the time of CEPI's inception, the Japanese government, with main donor countries as well as other organizations, pledged a financial contribution to this global partnership for the five years (Japan = 125 million dollars, Norway = 120 million dollars, Germany = 10.6 million dollars, Gates Foundation = 100 million dollars, Wellcome Trust = 100 million dollars).[7] It was arranged that the International Financial Facility for Immunization (IFFIm) would issue so-called "vaccine bonds" on behalf of CEPI, because IFFIm had both the global experience and expertise with credibility among international investors.

The establishment of CEPI provided opportunities of research and development (R&D) of vaccines and medicines in Japan as well, and on February 25, 2019, CEPI and the University of Tokyo announced

---

[5] This chapter is based on my earlier research on Japan and CEPI. See Akimoto, Daisuke. February 21, 2023. "Tokyo's Long View on the Coalition for Epidemic: The '100 Days Mission' and More". *ISDP Voices*. https://isdp.se/tokyos-long-view-on-the-coalition-for-epidemic-the-100-days-mission-and-more/.

[6] Ministry of Foreign Affairs of Japan. 2016. "G7 Ise-Shima Vision for Global Health". https://www.mofa.go.jp/files/000160273.pdf.

[7] Sun, Lena H. January 18, 2017. "New Global Coalition Launched to Create Vaccines, Prevent Epidemic". *Washington Post*. https://www.washingtonpost.com/news/to-your-health/wp/2017/01/18/new-global-coalition-launched-to-create-new-vaccines-prevent-epidemics/.

a "partnering agreement worth up to 31 million dollars to advance the development and manufacture of a vaccine against the Nipah virus".[8] In July 2019, it was announced that Japan's Dai-ichi Life Insurance Company had become a major purchaser of CEPI's vaccine bonds and IFFIm's first institutional investor in Japan.[9] In the face of the outbreak of coronavirus in China, CEPI announced it would fund vaccine development projects by the University of Queensland in Australia as well as Moderna on January 23, 2020.[10]

As a result of the global coalition for pandemic preparedness in cooperation with CEPI, vaccines for coronavirus were developed in 326 days after detection of the disease. This was the fastest in the history of vaccine development, thanks to the technology of mRNA vaccines.[11] Still, many people suffered and died of the coronavirus, and on March 10, 2021, CEPI set forth a "100 days mission" with a view to developing vaccines against new types of infectious diseases within 100 days after detection of the disease.[12]

The 100 days mission as a five-year program is designed to strengthen pandemic preparedness and global connection between different institutions, such as the Biomedical Advanced Research and Development Authority in the United States, the Health Emergency Preparedness and Response Authority in the European Union, and the Strategic Center of Biomedical Advanced Vaccine Research and Development for Preparedness and Response (SCARDA) of the Japan Agency for Medical

[8] CEPI. February 25, 2019. "CEPI Awards Contract Worth up to US$ 31 Million to the University of Tokyo to Develop Vaccine against Nipah Virus". https://cepi.net/news_cepi/cepi-awards-contract-worth-up-to-us-31-million-to-the-university-of-tokyo-to-develop-vaccine-against-nipah-virus/.

[9] IFFIm. July 18, 2019. "IFFIm Issues NOK600 Million Vaccine Bonds". https://iffim.org/press-releases/iffim-issues-nok600-million-vaccine-bonds.

[10] Coy, Peter. February 13, 2020. "The Road to a Coronavirus Vaccine Runs Through Oslo". *Bloomberg*. https://www.bloomberg.com/news/articles/2020-02-13/this-oslo-facility-may-be-the-key-to-the-coronavirus-vaccine?leadSource=uverify%20wall.

[11] NEC. 2022. "AI Technology Is Revolutionizing the Vaccine Development Industry". https://www.nec.com/en/global/sdgs/innovators/nvw2022/report.html.

[12] Kelland, Kate. March 10, 2021. "Coalition Eyes 100-Day Target for New Vaccines against Disease Epidemics". *Reuters*. https://www.reuters.com/article/us-health-coronavirus-vaccines-cepit-idUSKBN2B201K.

Research and Development in Japan, etc.[13] As a matter of fact, CEPI and SCARDA signed a memorandum of cooperation to "strengthen collaboration between the two organizations as they strive to accelerate global preparedness and response to future pandemics" on June 23, 2023.[14] In the midst of the COVID-19 pandemic, the Japanese government has regarded CEPI as indispensable for the swift development of vaccines and necessary preparedness for future pandemics.

## Domestic Supporter of CEPI: The Role of Komeito

With regards to the 100 days mission, CEPI estimated in March 2021 that 3.5 billion dollars would be necessary for pandemic preparedness activities and launched an investment case.[15] Meanwhile, Komeito as a coalition partner of the Liberal Democratic Party (LDP) has played a significant role in securing Japan's financial contribution to CEPI. To this end, Komeito has been actively engaged in support of CEPI as well as promotion of global health policy in Japan. On May 10, 2021, Seth Berkley as CEO of Gavi, the Vaccine Alliance, and CEPI CEO Richard Hatchett had an online meeting with Natsuo Yamaguchi, Chief Representative of Komeito.[16] Both Berkley and Hatchett commended Komeito for its role in facilitating Japan's participation in the COVAX Facility that contributed to the equal access of vaccines in developing countries. Especially, Hatchett asked Komeito to encourage the Japanese government to make a further financial contribution to the development of vaccines.

Notably, Bill Gates sent a letter of appreciation on June 9, 2021, to Komeito for the party's activities to strengthen Japan's commitment to global health, including CEPI. In the letter, Gates wrote "given Komeito's remarkable efforts in championing CEPI's work so far, the

---

[13] Lawler, Daniel. December 23, 2022. "Three Years into COVID-19: Are We Ready for the Next Pandemic?" *Japan Times*. https://www.japantimes.co.jp/news/2022/12/23/asia-pacific/three-years-covid-19-pandemic/.

[14] CEPI. June 26, 2023. "SCARDA and CEPI Collaborate to Strengthen Global Pandemic Preparedness and Response". https://cepi.net/news_cepi/scarda-and-cepi-collaborate-to-strengthen-global-pandemic-preparedness-and-response/.

[15] CEPI. 2021. "CEPI: 2022–2026 Strategy". https://cepi.net/wp-content/uploads/2021/03/20211201-CEPI-2022-2026-Strategy.pdf.

[16] Komei Shimbun. May 11, 2021. "Wakuchin Kyokyu Kobakkusu (Vaccine Supply through the COVAX Facility)".

party's role in reinforcing the collaboration between Japan and CEPI will become more important".[17] Furthermore, on February 15, 2022, the Global Health Promotion Committee of Komeito officially requested Shigeyuki Goto, Minister of Health, Labour and Welfare, to pledge additional 300 million dollars to CEPI for the next five years.[18] In response, Minister Goto responded that the ministry would like to coordinate this decision-making process so that Japan could take international responsibility for pandemic response and global health.[19] On November 24, 2022, Kaneshige Wakamatsu, a lawmaker of Komeito, asked Prime Minister Kishida if Japan would really intend to donate 300 million dollars to CEPI in the Committee on Health, Labour and Welfare of the Upper House. In response, Kishida reconfirmed the amount of the pledge to support CEPI's strategy.[20] Thus, Diet members of Komeito have consistently encouraged the Japanese government to support CEPI, playing an integral role in Japan's global health policy.

## THE 100 DAYS MISSION FOR FUTURE PANDEMICS

On February 25, 2022, Prime Minister Kishida held a teleconference with CEPI CEO Hatchett, and said that the Japanese government would pledge additional 300 million dollars to CEPI for the following five years, reaffirming that early development of and equitable access to vaccines are indispensable for strengthening global health security.[21] A statement by the Kishida administration noted that "Japan will strengthen its cooperation with CEPI to respond to the current pandemic and prepare for future pandemics. The contribution to CEPI has great significance in addressing the common human issue of pandemics and can also help to

[17] Komeito. June 17, 2021. "Gates Foundation Commends Komeito on COVAX Work". https://www.komei.or.jp/en/news/detail/20210617_28514.

[18] Komei Shimbun. February 17, 2022. "CEPI e Shikin Kyoshutsu ga Hitsuyo (Financial Support for CEPI Is Necessary)".

[19] Ibid.

[20] National Diet Library. November 24, 2022. "Proceedings of the 210th Diet Session, the Committee on Health, Labour and Welfare, the House of Councillors". https://kokkai.ndl.go.jp/txt/121014260X00820221124/27, https://kokkai.ndl.go.jp/txt/121014260X00820221124/28.

[21] Ministry of Health, Labour and Welfare. February 25, 2022. "Nihon kara Sepi ni Taisuru Aratana Kyoshutsu ni tsuite (Japan's Pledge on Additional Donation to CEPI)". https://www.mhlw.go.jp/stf/newpage_24098.html.

further promote Japan's own vaccine development and production. The government of Japan will continue to actively contribute to the development and production of vaccines for the international community".[22] With the additional pledge of 300 million dollars, Japan is the fourth largest donor country to CEPI in total (donations to CEPI 1.0 and CEPI 2.0) as shown in Fig. 11.1.[23]

In response to the decision by the Japanese government, Hatchett commended Japan, saying that "The government of Japan has long recognized and supported the imperative that no one is safe unless everyone is safe. Japan paved the way for the launch of CEPI with the 2016 G7 Ise-Shima Vision for Global Health and was one of CEPI's first funders. CEPI's success owes a great deal to the support of the Japanese

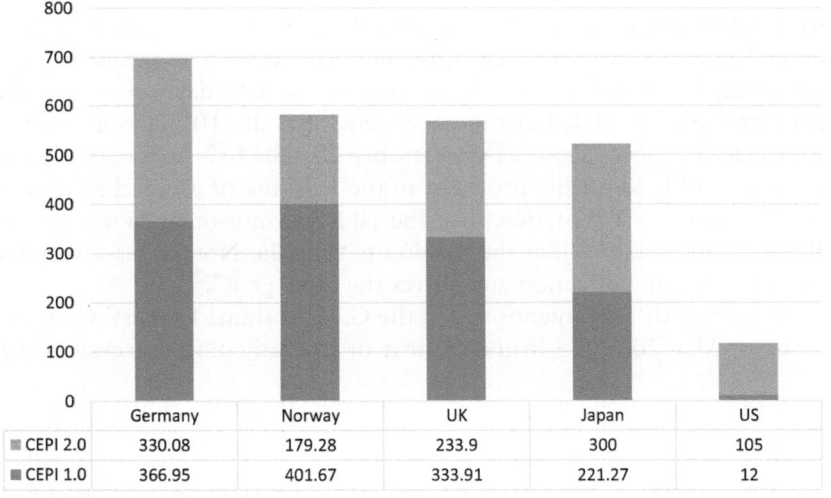

| | Germany | Norway | UK | Japan | US |
|---|---|---|---|---|---|
| CEPI 2.0 | 330.08 | 179.28 | 233.9 | 300 | 105 |
| CEPI 1.0 | 366.95 | 401.67 | 333.91 | 221.27 | 12 |

**Fig. 11.1** Top 5 donor countries to CEPI (CEPI 1.0 and CEPI 2.0) (*Note* Unit = US million dollars)

[22] CEPI. February 25, 2022. "Japan Pledges US$300 Million to CEPI's Pandemic Preparedness Plan". https://cepi.net/news_cepi/japan-pledges-us300-million-to-cepis-pandemic-preparedness-plan/.

[23] CEPI. December 1, 2023. "CEPI Investors Overview". https://100days.cepi.net/wp-content/uploads/2023/12/2023_12_01-CEPI-Investors-Overview.pdf.

people. We thank Prime Minister Fumio Kishida for this vital investment in the protection of the people of Japan, and the world, against future pandemics".[24] It is noteworthy that Hatchett recalled the 2016 G7 Ise-Shima Summit for CEPI's origins, recalling Japan's diplomatic contribution to the establishment of CEPI at the G7 summit.

Furthermore, Hatchett contributed an article to *Komei Shimbun*, published on January 14, 2023, encouraging the Japanese government to take leadership for global health at the G7 Hiroshima Summit.[25] In particular, Hatchett wrote: "CEPI is enormously grateful that Japan has embraced the 100 days mission as a critical pillar of its G7 Global Health agenda, and I am honored to be contributing to this agenda as an advisor to the G7 Global Health Task Force".[26] In addition to the political support by the Japanese government, NEC Corporation has collaborated with CEPI by making use of its artificial intelligence (AI) biotechnology to develop innovative vaccines against SARS-CoV-2 variants as well as other betacoronaviruses.[27] Thus, through the letter to a Japanese political party, CEPI stressed the significance of the 100 days mission in the pandemic period. Hatchett moreover reiterated the 100 days mission in an article of *Nikkei Shimbun* on October 22, 2022.[28] As for the significance of CEPI, Ken Ishii, professor of the Institute of Medical Science at the University of Tokyo, described the 100 days mission as "a mission for all humanity", stating that the mission is "like the North Star. Everyone looks in the same direction and shares the same goal".[29]

Notably, CEPI was mentioned in the G7 Hiroshima Leaders' Communique of May 20, 2023 in the context of strengthening universal health

[24] Ibid.

[25] Komeito. January 14, 2023. "CEPI CEO Calls for Japan, Komeito and G7 to Continue Fight against Infectious Diseases". https://www.komei.or.jp/en/news/detail/20230114_28726.

[26] Ibid.

[27] NEC. Aril 8, 2022. "CEPI Partners with Japan's NEC Group to Develop Artificial Intelligence-designed Broadly Protective Betacoronavirus Vaccine". https://www.nec.com/en/press/202204/global_20220408_02.html.

[28] Nikkei Shimbun. October 22, 2022. "100 Nichi de Wakuchin Sesshu Kyokyu Mezase (Let's Prepare for Vaccine Supply in the 100 Days)". https://www.nikkei.com/article/DGXZQOCB133940T11C22A0000000/.

[29] NHK. January 14, 2023. "Tech Firm Crunches Data for Next-gen Vaccine". https://www3.nhk.or.jp/nhkworld/en/news/backstories/2181/.

coverage (UHC) as well as global health architecture (GHA). It also referred to the 100 days mission as follows: "We reaffirm that innovative initiatives including those related to digital health are keys to strengthening GHA and achieving UHC. We will reiterate the urgent need to foster innovation and to strengthen research and development of safe, effective, quality-assured and affordable medical countermeasures (MCMs) as underlined by the 100 days mission".[30] Thus, the Japanese government has supported CEPI and the 100 days mission financially and diplomatically. In essence, Japan's contribution to CEPI will enhance the global health architecture as well as international framework for COVID-19 measures (ACT-A).[31] Having said that, Japan's total pledges and contributions to CEPI have been calculated as about 12.61 percent of all donor countries and groups as observed in *CEPI: 2022 Annual Progress Report*.[32] In other words, Japan as the fourth largest economy in the world is expected to make more financial and diplomatic contributions to CEPI as well as its 100 days mission in preparation for the next pandemic.

## Conclusion

This chapter has examined the importance of CEPI as a pandemic preparedness system, which was developed from the document of the G7 Ise-Shima Summit and discussed in the G7 Hiroshima Summit. As a host country of the G7 Hiroshima Summit, Japan highlighted the importance of global health. Japan is expected to make further contributions to pandemic preparedness and response to future pandemics, and hence, its continuous financial support for CEPI would be critical in the post-COVID-19 pandemic period. In this respect, the memorandum

---

[30] White House. May 20, 2023. "G7 Hiroshima Leaders' Communiqué". https://www.whitehouse.gov/briefing-room/statements-releases/2023/05/20/g7-hiroshima-leaders-communique/.

[31] Ezoe, Satoshi. 2021. "Toward New Solidarity in Global Health: Universal Health Coverage and Reform at the WHO". *Discuss Japan: Japan Foreign Policy Forum*. No. 67, pp. 1–7. https://www.japanpolicyforum.jp/pdf/2021/no67/DJweb_67_dip_02.pdf.

[32] CEPI. 2023. *CEPI: 2022 Annual Progress Report*. p. 78. https://cepi.net/wp-content/uploads/2023/06/CEPI-Annual-Progress-Report-2022.pdf.

of cooperation between CEPI and SCARDA will be of significance in preparation for "Disease X" in the future.[33]

It has also reconfirmed Japan's diplomatic contribution to the inception of CEPI at the G7 Ise-Shima Summit, the role of Komeito in facilitating Japan's global health policy on CEPI, and Japan's support for the 100 days mission that CEPI has been promoting in the coronavirus pandemic period. In particular, Diet members of Komeito officially requested the Japanese government to make financial contributions to CEPI, and made the prime minister reconfirm the amount of Japan's pledge to CEPI. It can be concluded that how the international community including Japan supports CEPI will determine how the human beings can prevent and prepare for future pandemics in the post-COVID-19 world.

[33] Embassy of Japan in the UK. June 23, 2023. "Remarks by H.E. Mr. HAYASHI Hajime, Ambassador of Japan to the UK, for Signature Ceremony of MOC between SCARDA and CEPI, Friday 23rd June 2023". https://www.uk.emb-japan.go.jp/itpr_ja/230623amb_00001.html.

# CHAPTER 12

# Conclusion: Japan, Global Health Actors, and the Global Health Architecture

**Abstract** Even in the anarchic nature of global politics, "global health governance" has existed, and "global health actors" have been committed to the function of the global health governance over decades. The key global health actors can be regarded as components of "global health architecture" in the global health system. This chapter sheds light on Japan and the global health architecture in reference to "special drawing rights" (SDRs) of the International Monetary Fund (IMF) as an example of one of the significant actors of the global health architecture in the post-COVID-19 pandemic world. Finally, this concluding chapter summarizes the key arguments and findings of previous chapters by reconfirming Japan's contributions to global health security and the implications for enhancing the global health architecture.

**Keywords** Coronavirus (COVID-19) · Global health actors · Global health governance · International Monetary Fund (IMF) · Japan · Special drawing rights (SDRs)

In the field of global politics, the nature of the international community is described as "anarchy", where the world government does not exist, but it does not mean that the nature of the world system is "disorder". If anything, there exists international order in this anarchical society.[1] Likewise, "global health governance" has existed as "a series of rules, norms and principles, some formal others less so, which are generally accepted by the key actors involved".[2] Indeed, global health actors have been committed to the function of the global health governance over decades,[3] and the key global health actors can be regarded as components of "global health architecture" in this anarchic world health system.

This chapter sheds light on Japan and the global health architecture in reference to "special drawing rights" (SDRs) of the International Monetary Fund (IMF) as an example of one of the significant actors of the global health architecture in the post-COVID-19 pandemic world. As a matter of fact, the IMF has contributed to the improvement of the global health system, and preventable diseases and disparities of longevity around the world should be rectified in the global health scene.[4] For example, it pays attention to the SDRs by the IMF in the middle of the coronavirus pandemic, while pointing out the aspect that there has been humanitarian crisis in Afghanistan in the meanwhile. Finally, this chapter summarizes the key arguments of this book by reconfirming Japan's contributions to global health and the implications for enhancing the global health architecture.[5]

[1] Bull, Hedley. 1977. *The Anarchical Society: A Study of Order in World Politics.* London: Macmillan.

[2] McInnes, Colin and Kelly Lee. 2012. *Global Health and International Relations.* Cambridge: Polity Press, p. 101.

[3] Shiroyama, Hideaki, ed. 2020. *Global Health Governance.* Tokyo: Toshindo Publishing.

[4] Bloom, David E. 2014. "The Shape of Global Health". IMF Finance and Development. https://www.imf.org/external/pubs/ft/fandd/2014/12/pdf/bloom.pdf.

[5] The chapter is partly based on my earlier research on Japan and IMF's SDRs. See, Akimoto, Daisuke. December 2, 2021. "Japan's Response to IMF's Special Drawing Rights in the COVID-19 Pandemic". *ISDP Voices.* https://www.isdp.eu/japans-response-to-imfs-special-drawing-rights-in-the-covid-19-pandemic/.

## IMF's Special Drawing Rights (SDRs) in the COVID-19 Pandemic

On August 2, 2021, the Board of Governors of the International Monetary Fund (IMF) approved a general allocation of Special Drawing Rights (SDRs) as international reserve assets equivalent to 650 billion dollars to boost global economic liquidity affected by the COVID-19 pandemic.[6] The new SDR allocation became effective on August 23, 2021. IMF Managing Director Kristalina Georgieva stated that "This is a historic decision – the largest SDR allocation in the history of the IMF and a shot in the arm for the global economy at a time of unprecedented crisis... It will particularly help our most vulnerable countries struggling to cope with the impact of the COVID-19 crisis".[7]

The SDR system was created in 1969 as a supplementary international reserve asset in the Bretton Woods fixed exchange rate system. The IMF decided to create and allocate SDRs as a supplemental reserve asset because the credibility of the US dollar was undermined by the United States' continuing trade deficit. Even after the collapse of the Bretton Woods system in 1973, SDRs have played a role as a global reserve asset— often referred to as "helicopter money",[8] a term originally coined by US economist Milton Friedman.[9] Moreover, it has been considered that the helicopter money is not necessarily distributed to low-income countries that need SDRs the most, as SDR allocation for IMF member countries is determined by their investment amount.

As a matter of fact, the IMF ruled out Afghanistan from the list of the general allocation of the SDRs because of an approval issue for the

---

[6] Heath, Michael. August 23, 2021. "IMF Urges $650b SDR Injection Be Directed to Covid's Hardest Hit". *Bloomberg*. https://www.bloomberg.com/news/articles/2021-08-23/imf-urges-650b-sdr-injection-be-directed-to-covid-s-hardest-hit.

[7] Ibid.

[8] Jones, Marc. April 7, 2009. "ECB's Stark Raps Move to Boost IMF Drawing Rights". *Reuters*. https://jp.reuters.com/article/uk-ecb-stark-sb/ecbs-stark-raps-move-to-boost-imf-drawing-rights-idUKTRE5362AQ20090407/.

[9] Economic Times. April 12, 2020. "ET Explains: What Is Helicopter Money and Why Is It in News?" https://economictimes.indiatimes.com/news/et-explains/what-is-helicopter-money-and-why-is-it-in-news/articleshow/75106564.cms?utm_source=contentofinterest&utm_medium=text&utm_campaign=cppst.

new Taliban administration.[10] Nevertheless, the economic situation in Afghanistan has been deteriorating, and it was reported on November 9, 2021, that at least 25 children in the Indira Gandhi Children's Hospital in Kabul passed away due to hunger and malnutrition.[11] According to the World Food Programme, as many as 45 million people in 43 countries are in danger of famine, and reportedly, the case of Afghanistan is the worst among them. The case of Afghanistan indicates that proper SDR allocation for the sake of vulnerable people is not an easy decision in certain political situations.[12]

The Chinese yuan, or Renminbi (RMB), was officially integrated into the SDR basket with the US dollar, Euro, Pound sterling, and Japanese yen in 2016.[13] It signifies that SDRs could be utilized within the framework of the Asian Infrastructure Investment Bank (AIIB) and the Silk Road Fund, operated in support of China's Belt and Road Initiative (BRI). IMF member states can utilize SDR not only for poverty reduction or medical and healthcare system improvements but also for multiple other purposes. Regarding this point, former Japanese Finance Minister Taro Aso warned that "There would be no point to it if SDR expansion is used for paying back debts to China".[14]

In the 44th meeting of the International Monetary and Financial Committee held in Washington on October 14, 2021, Japanese Finance Minister Shunichi Suzuki expressed an official statement and welcomed the new SDR allocation of 650 billion dollars. He stated that the Japanese government would "contribute to SDR channeling that utilizes the newly

[10] Martin, Eric. August 19, 2021. "IMF Curbs Afghanistan's Funding Access, Squeezing Taliban". *Bloomberg.* https://www.bloomberg.com/news/articles/2021-08-18/imf-says-afghanistan-can-t-access-sdrs-or-fund-s-resources.

[11] ABC News. November 9, 2021. "Afghanistan Children Suffer with Malnutrition as Unpaid Doctors and Taliban Bosses Clash in Hospitals". https://www.abc.net.au/news/2021-11-09/afghanistan-children-suffer-in-hospital-unpaid-doctors-taliban/100606902.

[12] Keath, Lee. November 9, 2021. "Emaciated Children in Kabul Hospital Underscore Rising Hunger in Afghanistan". *The Diplomat.* https://thediplomat.com/2021/11/emaciated-children-in-kabul-hospital-underscore-rising-hunger-in-afghanistan/.

[13] Goodman, Matthew P., Ye Yuand Daniel Remler. September 22, 2017. "Parallel Perspectives on the Global Economic Order". *CSIS Report.* https://www.csis.org/analysis/parallel-perspectives-global-economic-order.

[14] Kajimoto, Tetsushi. April 6, 2021. "Japan Backs New IMF Allocation, U.S. Calls for Minimum Corp Tax". *Reuters.* https://www.reuters.com/article/us-g20-debt-japan-idUSKBN2BT08I/.

allocated SDRs to support vulnerable countries, particularly low-income ones".[15] In concrete terms, the government would continue to make financial contributions to the Poverty Reduction and Growth Trust and support the IMF's proposal to create the Resilience and Sustainability Trust to address medium-term and long-term structural challenges, such as climate change and pandemic preparedness.

It is also possible for Japan as well as other G20 member countries to distribute the allocated SDRs through channels of multilateral development banks (MDBs), such as the World Bank and the Asia Development Bank.[16] The SDR allocation is not a cure-all solution for the global economy damaged by the coronavirus pandemic. Still, the balanced reallocation of the SDRs based on the three options above would be able to mitigate the danger for vulnerable people at risk of famine and malnutrition in the middle of the COVID-19 pandemic. In particular, children in Afghanistan are innocent and should not have to suffer from famine and malnutrition.

Japan's postwar economic recovery and rapid growth profoundly owed to the financial assistance by the World Bank and especially the International Bank for Reconstruction and Development (IBRD), which financed 31 projects in postwar Japan.[17] In this sense, Japan is responsible for making further financial contributions to the post-pandemic recovery of the global economy and suffering people in the post-COVID-19 world. Either way, it can be observed that the IMF in cooperation with the MDBs have been expected to make tremendous and continuous contributions to the poverty reduction and the improvement of the global health system.

---

[15] Ministry of Finance. October 14, 2021. "Statement by the Honorable SUZUKI Shunichi Governor of the IMF for Japan at the Forty-Fourth Meeting of the International Monetary and Financial Committee". https://www.mof.go.jp/english/policy/international_policy/imf/imfc/imfc_20211014_2.pdf.

[16] Andrews, David and Mark Plant. October 12, 2021. "Rechanneling SDRs to MDBs: Urgent Action Is Needed to Jumpstart the Green Equitable Transition". Center for Global Development. https://www.cgdev.org/blog/rechanneling-sdrs-mdbs-urgent-action-needed-jumpstart-green-equitable-transition.

[17] World Bank. September 17, 2020. "The World Bank in Japan". https://www.worldbank.org/en/country/japan/overview#1.

## Japan, Global Health Actors, and the Global Heath Architecture

From the perspective of the global health politics,[18] this book has examined Japan's global health policy in the pre-and post-COVID-19 pandemic era. It has investigated the role of global health actors, such as the COVAX Facility, Gavi, the Vaccine Alliance (Gavi), the Global Fund to Fight AIDS, Tuberculosis and Malaria (Global Fund), the Global Polio Eradication Initiative (GPEI), the Global Financing Facility for Women, Children and Adolescents (GFF), the Global Health Innovative Technology Fund (GHIT Fund), and the Coalition for Epidemic Preparedness Innovations (CEPI). It is fair to argue that all of them are components of the global health architecture. Moreover, this book has paid attention to Japan's contributions to the global health security through the Tokyo International Conference on African Development (TICAD) conferences and its ODA diplomacy.

It also scrutinized the role of the Business Leaders' Coalition for Global Health facilitated by the Bill & Melinda Gates Foundation (Gates Foundation) as well as leaders of Japanese companies. Furthermore, this chapter has examined Japan and the role of the IMF in the middle of the coronavirus pandemic. Generally, it is fair to argue that they are all "global health actors". Still, what exactly are global health actors? Broadly speaking, global health actors can be divided into the three groups: "bilateral donors, multilaterals donors, and non-governmental agencies and increasingly the private sector".[19] More specifically however, the global health actors as components of the global health architecture can be categorized as Table 12.1.[20]

---

[18] McInnes, Colin, Kelley Lee, and Jeremy Youde, eds. 2020. *The Oxford Handbook of Global Health Politics*. Oxford: Oxford University Press.

[19] Soucat, Agnès and Richard Gregory. 2022. "Understanding the Global Health Architecture". In Siddiqi, Sameen, Awad Mataria, Katherine D. Rouleau, and Meesha Iqbal, eds. 2022. *Making Health Systems Work in Low and Middle Income Countries: Textbook for Public Health Practitioners*. Cambridge: Cambridge University Press, pp. 545–562.

[20] Gostin, Lawrence O., Eric A. Friedman, and Alexandra Finch. August 4, 2023. "The Global Health Architecture: Governance and International Institutions to Advance Population Health Worldwide". *Milbank Quarterly*. Vol. 101. No. S1: Special Centennial Issue: The Future of Population Health: Challenges & Opportunities, pp. 734–769. https://papers.ssrn.com/sol3/papers.cfm?abstract_id=4434217.

**Table 12.1** Global health actors as components of the global health architecture

| Category of organizations | Names of global health actors |
| --- | --- |
| UN Organs | UN General Assembly, UN Security Council |
| UN Agencies, Funds, etc. | WHO, UNDP, FAO, UNAIDS, IMF, UNICEF, etc. |
| Multilateral Organizations | OECD (DAC), WTO, World Bank Group, etc. |
| Intergovernmental Forums | G7 and G20, the Quad (vaccine partnership), etc. |
| Government Organs | Ministries and Agencies (MOFA, MHLW, MOF, etc.) |
| Public–Private Partnerships | Global Fund, Gavi, Unitaid, CEPI, GPEI, GFF, GHIT, etc. |
| Philanthropic Organizations | Bill & Melinda Gates Foundation, Wellcome Trust, etc. |
| Civil Society Organizations | MSF, Save the Children Japan, Results Japan, JCIE etc. |
| Academic Institutions | Japan Association for Global Health, universities, etc. |
| Companies and coalitions | Business Leaders' Coalition for Global Health, etc. |
| Medical Service Workers | Doctors and nurses at hospitals and clinics, GHEC, etc. |

*Note* Created by the author based on previous chapters in reference to Lawrence, Friedman, and Finch (2023)

Global health architecture is defined as "the relationship between the many different actors engaged in global health and the processes through which they work together".[21] In this sense, previous chapters have traced the role of the global health actors as well as the development of the global health architecture in the both pre-and post-COVID-19 world. In Chapter 1, Japan and global health issues have been analyzed in the context of the coronavirus pandemic. It examined the development of Japan's human security diplomacy by paying attention to Prime Minister Abe's epistemic contributions to *Lancet*. Then, Japan's commitments to the COVID-19 pandemic have been discussed as an example of emerging Japan's new global health strategy based on its human security diplomacy. In Chapter 2, Japan's diplomatic contributions to the entry into the COVID-19 Vaccines Global Access (COVAX) Facility toward a more equal distribution of coronavirus vaccines in the world. It investigated

[21] Sakamoto, Haruka, Satoshi Ezoe, Kotono Hara, Yui Sekitani, Keishi Abe, Haruhiko Inada, Takuma Kato, Kenichi Komada, Masami Miyakawa, Eiji Hinoshita, Hiroyuki Yamaya, Naoko Yamamoto, Sarah Krull Abe, and Kenji Shibuya. 2018. "Japan's Contribution to Making Global Health Architecture a Top Political Agenda by Leveraging the G7 Presidency". *Journal of Global Health*. Vol. 8, No. 2. https://www.ncbi.nlm.nih.gov/pmc/articles/PMC6269922/.

Japan's contributions to Gavi and the COVAX Facility in terms of both domestic and external factors. It shed light on the role of Komeito as a ruling party that had strenuously facilitated Japan's global health policy as well as Japan's entry into the COVAX Facility. Then, Japan's financial contributions to the COVAX Facility have been scrutinized as well as its diplomatic implications for the free and open Indo-Pacific (FOIP) vision.

Chapter 3 examined Japan's contributions to the Global Fund. It contextualized the significance of the G8 Kyushu-Okinawa Summit as an origin of establishing the Global Fund. It reconfirmed that Japan's policy toward the Global Fund has been multi-partisan including both ruling and opposition parties. Then, it warned that health system in Ukraine was devastated and the humanitarian situations in war-torn Ukraine should not be forgotten by the international community, especially the G7 countries, in the middle of the ongoing Russia-Ukraine War. Chapter 4 shed light of Japan's contributions to the GPEI as well as the two polio endemic countries, namely Afghanistan and Pakistan. It contextualized that Japan overcame wild poliovirus in the country and adopted the IPV. It moreover analyzed the human development index (HDI) of Afghanistan and Pakistan as well as Japan's bilateral financial contributions to the two endemic countries. It concluded that Japan should make more financial contributions not only to the two poliovirus endemic countries but also to the GPEI toward a polio-free world.

Chapter 5 provided an analysis on the development of Japan's human security diplomacy toward Africa through the examination of TICAD conferences. The chapter confirmed that Japan has made consistent contributions to the development of Africa, and an emphasis on global health has been strengthened especially in the pandemic period. It also examined Japan's motivations toward TICAD diplomacy in terms of both realist and liberal perspectives. TICAD 8 witnessed Prime Minister Kishida's pledge of 1.08 billion dollars to the Global Fund, symbolizing Japan's contributions to human security and global health in Africa. It has been observed that Japan is expected to make a further contribution toward the 2025 TICAD 9. Chapter 6 paid attention to Japan's changing ODA diplomacy in the light of global health politics. As discussed in the chapter, Japan's ODA policy has been shaped based on both national interests and humanitarian purposes. In the Cold War period, Japan's ODA policy was influenced by the Cold War politics as well as its war reparation processes. It was confirmed that the 2003 ODA Charter adopted the aspect of national interests and the 2015 Development Cooperation Chater enabled Japan to provide ODA with foreign military forces for non-military purposes. Significantly, the 2023 Development Cooperation Charter reflected on the significance of global health as part of Japan's ODA strategy in the pandemic period.

Chapter 7 investigated the Japanese Business Leaders' Coalition for Global Health. Notably, the Bill & Melinda Gates Foundation has played an indispensable role in the global health promotion movement. Moreover, the chapter has clarified that Japanese companies, such as NEC, Shionogi, Daiwa Securities, Toyota Tsusho, Yamaha Motor, miup, and Sora Technology, have been committed to the improvement of global health in the world. The 2022 Global Health Action Japan exemplified the political influence of the business leaders' coalition over the decision-makers in Japan. In addition, a series of Global Health Academy organized by the business leaders' coalition were examined as substantial contributions to the field of global health in Japan and the world. It became evident that the Japanese business leaders have made incremental contributions to the promotion of Japan's global health policy behind the scene. Chapter 8 highlighted Japan's diplomatic and financial contributions to the GFF. The chapter has revealed that the Japanese government has made continucus commitments to the GFF from its initiation to the present. Since nutrition and health of mothers and children are integral part of global health, Japan's further contributions to the GFF would be integral for the improvement of global health around the globe.

Chapter 9 shed light on neglected tropical diseases (NTDs) which literally tend to be neglected in the middle of the coronavirus pandemic period. It reviewed Japan's commitments to the NTDs both domestically and externally. In particular, the chapter dealt with dengue fever, Hansen's disease, and lymphatic filariasis as examples of Japan's successful contributions to the control and eradication of the NTDs in the country. Importantly, the chapter clarified the role of the GHIT Fund as Japan's initiative as global health policy. It proposed that impact of the GHIT can be visualized with measurable data so that the future investment in the GHIT can be sustainable and meaningful. Chapter 10 briefly reviewed Japan's global health strategy toward the G7 Hiroshima Summit while investigating Japan's summit diplomacy as a host nation of G7/G8. It pointed out that the Pandemic Treaty as well as non-first use of nuclear weapons could have been deliberated in the diplomatic endeavors as agenda items of global health. Chapter 11 touched on the role of CEPI and Japan's support for the 100 days mission promoted by CEPI. The chapter reconfirmed that Japan has made diplomatic and financial contributions to CEPI. It became clear that Japan's global health policy includes not only disease control and eradication but also preparation for future pandemics. Finally, this chapter has discussed the role of the IMF in the poverty reduction and the global health system. Japan's financial contribution to the IMF's SDRs should be redistributed for the sake of the strengthening of the global health architecture in the pandemic world.

All these chapters have assisted in identifying global health actors as well as the existence of the global health architecture, which has been shaped and strengthened by global health governance. As argued by Kayo Takuma as a professor of Tokyo Metropolitan University, Japan has led the global health governance,[22] by cooperating with other global health actors and enhancing the global health architecture. In Japan, the Center on Global Health Architecture was established in Mitsubishi UFJ Research and Consulting with a view to connecting Japanese firms with international organizations so that Japanese companies would be able to make contributions to the field of global health.[23] Nonetheless, the center intends to provide consulting service with Japanese business leaders regarding international procurement in the field of global health, and they do not necessarily provide academic observation or analysis. Globally, the World Health Organization (WHO) has attempted to strengthen the global health architecture in terms of "health promotion (prevention of diseases), primary health care (as the foundation of universal health coverage), and health security (health emergency preparedness, response and resilience)".[24] Without a doubt, the WHO has played an integral role in shaping and enhancing the global health architecture.

Meanwhile, some Japanese lawmakers have discussed the importance of establishing and enhancing the global health architecture at the National Diet. On March 23, 2016, Keizo Takemi of the Liberal Democratic Party

---

[22] Takuma, Kayo. September 30, 2020. "Japan Leading Global Health Governance". *East Asia Forum.* https://www.eastasiaforum.org/2020/09/30/japan-leading-global-health-governance/.

[23] MUFJ Research and Consulting. 2023. "Center on Global Health Architecture". https://www.globalhealth.murc.jp/globalhealth/architecture/index.html.

[24] World Health Organization (WHO). May 23, 2022. "Strengthening the Global Architecture for Health Emergency Preparedness, Response and Resilience". https://apps.who.int/gb/ebwha/pdf_files/WHA75/A75_20-en.pdf.

(LDP) asked Yasuhisa Shiozaki, Minister of Health, Labour and Welfare, whether Japan would plan to contribute to global health at the G7 Ise-Shima Summit and the TICAD. In response, Minister Shiozaki pointed out the significance of attaining universal health coverage (UHC) on a global scale, and argued that Japan should show how the international community should create the global health architecture at the event of the G7 Ise-Shima Summit.[25]

Takemi and Shiozaki brought the issue of the global health architecture at the Diet from time to time, and it was included as one of the agenda items of the G7 Ise-Shima Summit. In the G7 Ise-Shima Leaders' Declaration, "reinforcing of the global health architecture to strengthen response to public health emergencies" was stipulated as one of the main issues of global health. The communique declared that the G7 countries would take leadership in reinforcing the global health architecture by supporting and strengthening the existing organizations, such as the WHO. Importantly, the G7 communique called on the international community to support the "Contingency Fund for Emergency" and welcomed the launching of the "Pandemic Emergency Financing Facility" formally announced by the World Bank.[26]

Japan's diplomatic contributions to strengthening the global health architecture was demonstrated again at the G7 Hiroshima Summit as well. Indeed, the G7 Hiroshima Leaders' Communique reads "We renew our strong commitment to developing and strengthening the global health architecture (GHA) with the World Health Organization (WHO) at its core for future public health emergencies to break the cycle of panic and neglect, recognizing that the COVID-19 pandemic has made an unprecedented impact on the international community".[27] The communique also expressed that the G7 countries would collaborate with the

---

[25] National Diet Library. March 23, 2016. "Proceedings of the 190th Diet Session. Committee on Health, Labour and Welfare, the House of Councillors". https://kokkai.ndl.go.jp/txt/119014260X00820160323/23, https://kokkai.ndl.go.jp/txt/119014260X00820160323/24.

[26] Ministry of Foreign Affairs of Japan. May 26–27, 2016. "G7 Ise-Shima Leaders' Declaration G7 Ise-Shima Summit, 26–27 May 2016". https://www.mofa.go.jp/files/000160266.pdf.

[27] Ministry of Foreign Affairs of Japan. May 20, 2023. "G7 Hiroshima Leaders' Communiqué", p. 22. https://www.mofa.go.jp/files/100506907.pdf.

"G20 Joint Finance and Health Task Force" and welcomed the launch of the Pandemic Fund.[28]

The communique moreover mentioned "the importance of strengthening and maintaining sufficient and high-quality human resources for health worldwide at all times, such as the public health and emergency workforce including consideration of Global Health Emergency Corps".[29] Incidentally, the idea of establishing the Global Health Emergency Corps (GHEC) was first proposed by Bill Gates in 2022,[30] and it would constitute a critical part of the global health architecture in the post-COVID-19 pandemic world. As illustrated in Japan's Global Health Strategy, the global health architecture is "a system for global cooperation and collaboration" based on UHC, and Japan has made consistent contributions to the strengthening of the global health architecture.[31] As investigated in this concluding chapter, a variety of global health actors have been involved in composing the global health architecture. This research has therefore substantiated that Japan has made continuous commitments and contributions to the establishment and improvement of the global health architecture in collaboration with other global health actors during the pre-and post-COVID-19 pandemic world.

[28] Ibid.

[29] Ibid., p. 23.

[30] Morrison, J. Stephen. August 31, 2023. "Dr. Scott Dowell, the Bill & Melinda Gates Foundation: 'I Am Optimistic'". Center for Strategic & International Studies (CSIS). https://www.csis.org/podcasts/commonhealth/dr-scott-dowell-bill-melinda-gates-foundation-i-am-optimistic.

[31] Prime Minister of Japan and His Cabinet. May 24, 2022. "Global Health Strategy of Japan", pp. 4 and 8. https://www.kantei.go.jp/jp/singi/kenkouiryou/en/pdf/final_GHS.pdf.

# Bibliography

ABC News. November 9, 2021. "Afghanistan Children Suffer with Malnutrition as Unpaid Doctors and Taliban Bosses Clash in Hospitals". https://www.abc.net.au/news/2021-11-09/afghanistan-children-suffer-in-hospital-unpaid-doctors-taliban/100606902.

Abe, Shinzo. September 14, 2013. "Japan's Strategy for Global Health Diplomacy: Why It Matters". *Lancet*. Vol. 382, No. 9896, pp. 915–916.

Abe, Shinzo. December 12, 2015. "Japan's Vision for a Peaceful and Healthier World". *Lancet*. Vol. 386, No. 10011, pp. 2367–2369.

African Union. 2012. "The African Peace and Security Architecture (APSA)". https://www.peaceau.org/en/topic/the-african-peace-and-security-architecture-apsa.

African Union. 2020. "Campaign for Accelerated Reduction of Maternal Mortality in Africa (CARMMA) 2009–2019". https://au.int/en/pressreleases/20200206/campaign-accelerated-reduction-maternal-mortality-africa-carmma-2009-2019.

African Development Bank. August 26, 2022. "Abe's Legacy in Africa under Scrutiny at Development Summit". https://www.afdb.org/en/news-and-events/abes-legacy-africa-under-scrutiny-development-summit-54367.

AIDS Prevention Information Network. 2020. "Annual Report on AIDS 2020". https://api-net.jfap.or.jp/status/japan/data/2020/nenpo/bunseki.pdf.

Akimoto, Daisuke May 6, 2020. "COVID-19 and Japan's Global Health Strategy: Developing Vaccines in a Human Security Crisis". *ISDP Voices*. https://isdp.eu/covid-19-japans-global-health-strategy/.

Akimoto, Daisuke. 2021. "The Clash of Japan's FOIP and China's BRI?" *Journal of Politics and Development (The REST)*. Vol. 11, No. 2, pp. 88–99.

Akimoto, Daisuke. December 2, 2021. "Japan's Response to IMF's Special Drawing Rights in the COVID-19 Pandemic". *ISDP Voices*. https://www.isdp.eu/japans-response-to-imfs-special-drawing-rights-in-the-covid-19-pandemic/.

Akimoto, Daisuke. December 28, 2021. "The Gates-Kishida Talks and Japan's New 'Global Health Strategy'". *The Diplomat*. https://thediplomat.com/2021/12/the-gates-kishida-talks-and-japans-new-global-health-strategy/.

Akimoto, Daisuke. 2022. *Japanese Prime Ministers and Their Peace Philosophy: 1945 to the Present*. Singapore: Palgrave Macmillan.

Akimoto, Daisuke. December 2022. "Japan Leads the Way in Global Health Diplomacy: The Case of Neglected Tropical Diseases (NTDs)". *ISDP Issue Brief*, pp. 1–9.

Akimoto, Daisuke. February 10, 2022. "Japan's Changing ODA Diplomacy". *The Diplomat*. https://thediplomat.com/2022/02/japans-changing-oda-diplomacy/.

Akimoto, Daisuke. March 31, 2022. "TICAD: The Evolution of Japan's Africa Diplomacy". *The Diplomat*. https://thediplomat.com/2022/03/ticad-the-evolution-of-japans-africa-diplomacy/.

Akimoto, Daisuke. April 21, 2022. "Japan's Vaccine Diplomacy toward a 'Polio-Free' World". *ISDP Voices*. https://isdp.eu/japans-vaccine-diplomacy-toward-a-polio-free-world/.

Akimoto, Daisuke. June 2, 2022. "Japan's Diplomatic Commitment to the Global Fund". *ISDP Voices*. https://www.isdp.eu/japan-committed-to-support-global-fund/.

Akimoto, Daisuke. July 12, 2022. "Japan's Global Health Diplomacy and the COVAX Facility". *ISDP Voices*. https://www.isdp.eu/japans-global-health-diplomacy-and-the-covax-facility/.

Akimoto, Daisuke. August 30, 2022. "Japan's Incrementalism in the World Bank's Global Financing Facility". *ISDP Voices*. https://isdp.eu/japans-incrementalism-in-the-world-banks-global-financing-facility/.

Akimoto, Daisuke. September 21, 2022. "Japan's Global Health Strategy: A Diplomatic Foresight on the G7 Hiroshima Summit". *ISDP Voices*. https://isdp.eu/japans-global-health-strategy-a-diplomatic-foresight-on-the-g7-hiroshima-summit/.

Daisuke Akimoto. November 5, 2022. "Human Security Agenda in Japan's Global Health Strategy in the COVID-19 Pandemic Era". Presentation at the Japan Association for Human Security Studies Annual Conference 2022. https://jahss2022.wixsite.com/mysite/day1.

Akimoto, Daisuke. February 21, 2023. "Tokyo's Long View on the Coalition for Epidemic: The '100 Days Mission' and More". *ISDP Voices*. https://isdp.se/tokyos-long-view-on-the-coalition-for-epidemic-the-100-days-mission-and-more/.

Akiyama, Shinichi. April 4, 2020. "US Embassy in Japan Urges Citizens to Return Home, Citing Lack of Virus Testing". *Mainichi Shimbun*. https://mainichi.jp/english/articles/20200404/p2a/00m/0in/014000c.

Aljazeera. March 14, 2023. "Taliban Launches Annual Polio Vaccination Drive in Afghanistan". https://www.aljazeera.com/news/2023/3/14/taliban-launches-annual-polio-vaccination-drive-in-afghanistan.

Amakasu Raposo, Pedro. 2014. *Japan's Foreign Aid Policy in Africa Evaluating the TICAD Process*. New York: Palgrave.

Amakasu Raposo, Pedro. 2014. *Japan's Foreign Aid to Africa: Angola and Mozambique Within the TICAD Process*. New York: Routledge.

Andrews, David and Mark Plant. October 12, 2021. "Rechanneling SDRs to MDBs: Urgent Action Is Needed to Jumpstart the Green Equitable Transition". Center for Global Development. https://www.cgdev.org/blog/rechanneling-sdrs-mdbs-urgent-action-needed-jumpstart-green-equitable-transition.

Asahi Shimbun. August 8, 2022. "U.N. Chief Urges Nuke Powers to Abide by No-First-Use Pledge". https://www.asahi.com/ajw/articles/14690104.

Asian Scientist. September 27, 2019. "Asia's Scientific Trailblazers: Catherine Ohura". https://www.asianscientist.com/2019/09/features/asias-scientific-trailblazers-catherine-ohura-ghit-fund/.

Bangkok Post. April 1, 2020. "Japan's Fujifilm Starts Avigan Trial to Treat Coronavirus". https://www.bangkokpost.com/world/1890935/japans-fujifilm-starts-avigan-trial-to-treat-coronavirus.

Barber, Harriet. March 5, 2022. "War in Ukraine Could Lead to 'Devastating' Tuberculosis Problem, Warns Anthony Fauci". *The Telegraph*. https://www.telegraph.co.uk/global-health/science-and-disease/war-ukraine-could-lead-devastating-tuberculosis-problem-warns/.

Bloom, David E. 2014. "The Shape of Global Health". IMF Finance and Development. https://www.imf.org/external/pubs/ft/fandd/2014/12/pdf/bloom.pdf.

Bull, Hedley. 1977. *The Anarchical Society: A Study of Order in World Politics*. London: Macmillan.

Butler, Declan. 2017. "Billion-Dollar Project Aims to Prep Vaccines Before Epidemics Hit". *Nature*. Vol. 541, No. 7638, pp. 444–445.

Cabinet Office, Japan. March 26, 2008. "On Malaria". https://www.cao.go.jp/noguchisho/award/maraliafact.html.

Centers for Disease Control and Prevention (CDC). 2020. *Yellow Book 2020*. https://wwwnc.cdc.gov/travel/yellowbook/2020/travel-related-infectious-diseases/malaria.

Centers of Disease Control and Prevention (CDC). 2022. "Parasites: Lymphatic Filariasis". https://www.cdc.gov/parasites/lymphaticfilariasis/index.html.

Centers of Disease Control and Prevention (CDC). 2022. "Hansen's Disease (Leprosy)". https://www.cdc.gov/leprosy/index.html.

Centers of Disease Control and Prevention (CDC). 2022. "Dengue During Pregnancy". https://www.cdc.gov/dengue/transmission/pregnancy.html.

Centers of Disease Control and Prevention (CDC). 2022. "Neglected Tropical Diseases (NTDs)". https://www.cdc.gov/globalhealth/ntd/index.html.

CEPI. February 25, 2019. "CEPI Awards Contract Worth Up to US$ 31 Million to the University of Tokyo to Develop Vaccine against Nipah Virus". https://cepi.net/news_cepi/cepi-awards-contract-worth-up-to-us-31-million-to-the-university-of-tokyo-to-develop-vaccine-against-nipah-virus/.

CEPI. 2021. "CEPI: 2022–2026 Strategy". https://cepi.net/wp-content/uploads/2021/03/20211201-CEPI-2022-2026-Strategy.pdf.

CEPI. 2022. "COVAX: CEPI's Response to COVID-19". https://cepi.net/covax/.

CEPI. February 25, 2022. "Japan Pledges US$300 Million to CEPI's Pandemic Preparedness Plan". https://cepi.net/news_cepi/japan-pledges-us300-million-to-cepis-pandemic-preparedness-plan/.

CEPI. 2023. *CEPI: 2022 Annual Progress Report*. https://cepi.net/wp-content/uploads/2023/06/CEPI-Annual-Progress-Report-2022.pdf.

CEPI. 2023. "CEPI: Preparing for Future Pandemics". https://cepi.net.

CEPI. 2023. "CEPI: Priority Diseases". https://cepi.net/research_dev/priority-diseases/.

CEPI. June 26, 2023. "SCARDA and CEPI Collaborate to Strengthen Global Pandemic Preparedness and Response". https://cepi.net/news_cepi/scarda-and-cepi-collaborate-to-strengthen-global-pandemic-preparedness-and-response/.

CEPI. December 1, 2023. "CEPI Investors Overview". https://100days.cepi.net/wp-content/uploads/2023/12/2023_12_01-CEPI-Investors-Overview.pdf.

Clements, Kevin P. April 2020. "Confronting the Covid-19 Crisis: Danger and Opportunity". *Toda Peace Institute Director's Statement*. https://toda.org/assets/files/resources/policy-briefs/t-pb-71_kevin-clements_director-statement-on-covid-19.pdf.

Colombo Plan. 2022. "The Colombo Plan". https://colombo-plan.org.

Coy, Peter. February 13, 2020. "The Road to a Coronavirus Vaccine Runs Through Oslo". *Bloomberg*. https://www.bloomberg.com/news/articles/2020-02-13/this-oslo-facility-may-be-the-key-to-the-coronavirus-vaccine?leadSource=uverify%20wall.

Craig, Allen S., Rustam Haydarov, Helena O'Malley, Michael Galway, Halima Dao, Ngashi Ngongo, Marie Therese Baranyikwa, Savita Naqvi, Nima S. Abid, Carol Pandak, and Amy Edwards. 2017. "The Public Health Legacy of Polio Eradication in Africa". *Journal of Infectious Diseases*. Vol. 216, No. 1, pp. 343–350.

Daiwa Securities Group. 2020. "Daiwa Securities Group and SDGs". https://www.daiwa-grp.jp/english/sdgs/data/pdf/daiwa_sdgs_en_booklet_2020sec.pdf.

Dattani, Saloni, Fiona Spooner, Sophie Ochmann, and Max Roser. 2022. "Polio". *Our World in Data* (First published in November 2017 and last updated in April 2022). https://ourworldindata.org/polio.

de Campos, Rodrigo Pires and Saori Kawai. 2022. "Japan's ODA to Developing Countries in the Health Sector: Overall Trend and Future Prospects". In Hamaguchi, Nobuaki and Danielly Ramos, eds. 2022. *Brazil-Japan Cooperation: From Complementarity to Shared Value*. Singapore: Springer, pp. 43–83.

Donor Tracker. July 20, 2023. "Japan / Global Health: ODA Spending". https://donortracker.org/donor_profiles/japan/globalhealth.

Drugs for Neglected Diseases initiative (DNDi). 2022. "Drugs for Neglected Diseases initiative". https://dndi.org/.

Economic Times. April 12, 2020. "ET Explains: What Is Helicopter Money and Why Is It in News?" https://economictimes.indiatimes.com/news/et-explains/what-is-helicopter-money-and-why-is-it-in-news/articleshow/75106564.cms?utm_source=contentofinterest&utm_medium=text&utm_campaign=cppst.

Edström, Bert. 2010. "Japan and the TICAD Process". *ISDP Asia Paper*. https://isdp.eu/content/uploads/publications/2010_edstrom_japan-and-the-ticad.pdf.

Edström, Bert. March 2011. "Japan and Human Security: The Derailing of a Foreign Policy Vision". *ISDP Asia Paper*. https://isdp.eu/content/uploads/images/stories/isdp-main-pdf/2011_edstrom_japan-and-human-security.pdf.

Eisai. 2014. "History of Lymphatic Filariasis Elimination in Japan". https://atm.eisai.co.jp/english/activity/.

Eisai. November 15, 2022. "Request to Position 'Global Health' as a Major Pillar of the Next Development Cooperation Charter". https://www.eisai.com/sustainability/atm/ntds/activity/030.html.

Elahi, Ebby. 2020 *Insights in Global Health: A Compendium of Healthcare Facilities and Nonprofit Organizations*. Oxon: Taylor & Francis Group.

Embassy of Japan in the UK. June 23, 2023. "Remarks by H.E. Mr. HAYASHI Hajime, Ambassador of Japan to the UK, for Signature Ceremony of MOC between SCARDA and CEPI, Friday 23rd June 2023". https://www.uk.emb-japan.go.jp/itpr_ja/230623amb_00001.html.

Every Woman Every Child. 2016. "2020 Progress Report on the EWEC Global Strategy". https://www.everywomaneverychild.org.

Eyinla, Bolade M. 2018. "Promoting Japan's National Interest in Africa". *African Development*. Vol. 43, No. 3, pp. 107–122.

Ezoe, Satoshi. 2021. "Toward New Solidarity in Global Health: Universal Health Coverage and Reform at the WHO". *Discuss Japan: Japan Foreign Policy Forum*. No. 67, pp. 1–7. https://www.japanpolicyforum.jp/pdf/2021/no67/DJweb_67_dip_02.pdf.

Faculty of Tropical Medicine, Mahidol University. 2008. "50th Anniversary of the Faculty of Tropical Medicine, Mahidol University: History". https://www.tm.mahidol.ac.th/50th-anniversary/history.htm.

Fernandes, Genevie and Devi Sridhar. 2017. "World Bank and the Global Financing Facility". *BMJ*. Vol. 358, p. 3.

Friedman, Eric A., Lawrence O. Gostin, Matthew M. Kavanagh, John T. Monahan, and Harold Hongju Koh. September 15, 2020. "Joining COVAX Could Save American Lives". *Foreign Policy*. https://foreignpolicy.com/2020/09/15/covax-vaccine-covid-19-trump-save-lives-equitable-distribution/.

Friends of the Global Fund, Japan. August 3, 2022. "Ahead of the 7th Replenishment, Diet Task Force Members Submit a Letter to the Japanese Government Asking for a Strong Global Fund Pledge". https://fgfj.jcie.or.jp/en/news/diet-task-force-letter-2022/.

Fukushima, Akiko. April 16, 2020. "COVID-19 Is a Human Security Crisis". *East Asia Forum*. https://www.eastasiaforum.org/2020/04/16/covid-19-is-a-human-security-crisis/.

Gates, Bill. 2022. *How to Prevent the Next Pandemic*. New York: Knopf.

Gates, Bill. May 2022. "No More Pandemics". https://www.gatesnotes.com/How-to-Prevent-the-Next-Pandemic.

Gavi. 2022. "COVAX". https://www.gavi.org/covax-facility.

Gavi. April 8, 2022. "Break COVID Now". https://www.gavi.org/sites/default/files/covid/covax/Gavi-Break-COVID-Now-Summit-2022-Chairs-Summary.pdf.

Gavi. 2023. "About Our Alliance". https://www.gavi.org/our-alliance/about.

Gavi. 2023. "Donor Profiles: Japan (as of June 30, 2023)". https://www.gavi.org/investing-gavi/funding/donor-profiles/japan.

GHIT Fund. 2022. "Global Health Innovative Technology Fund". https://www.ghitfund.org.

GHIT Fund. 2022. "Funding Partners and Sponsors". https://www.ghitfund.org/overview/partners.

GHIT Fund. 2022. "GHIT Fund Annual Report 2021". https://www.ghitfund.org/assets/othermedia/annual_report_2021_eng.pdf.

GHIT Fund. 2023. "Investment Overview: Investment to Date Since 2013". https://www.ghitfund.org/investment/overview/jp.

Global Financing Facility (GFF). December 14, 2017. "Government of Japan to Invest US$50 Million in Global Financing Facility to Accelerate Progress on Universal Health Coverage". https://www.globalfinancingfacility.org/govern ment-japan-invest-us50-million-global-financing-facility-accelerate-progress-universal-health.

Global Financing Facility (GFF). 2022. "JICA". https://www.globalfinancingfac ility.org/japan-international-cooperation-agency.

Global Financing Facility (GFF). 2022. "Our Response to COVID-19". https://www.globalfinancingfacility.org/where-we-work.

Global Health Progress. 2020. "The London Declaration on NTDs". https://globalhealthprogress.org/collaboration/the-london-declaration-on-ntds-2/.

Global Polio Eradication Initiative (GPEI). 2021. "Contributions and Pledges to the Global Polio Eradication Initiative, 1985–2020". https://polioerad ication.org/wp-content/uploads/2021/07/GPEI_FIN_Historical-Contribut ions_Journals-Charts_asat_2020-12-31.pdf.

Global Polio Eradication Initiative (GPEI). July 13, 2022. "In Remembrance of the Former Prime Minister of Japan, Hon. Shinzo Abe". https://polioe radication.org/news-post/in-remembrance-of-the-former-prime-minister-of-japan-hon-shinzo-abe/.

Goodman, Brenda. July 22, 2022. "New York Adult Diagnosed with Polio, First US Case in Nearly a Decade". *CNN*. https://edition.cnn.com/2022/07/21/health/new-york-polio/index.html.

Goodman, Matthew P., Ye Yuand Daniel Remler. September 22, 2017. "Parallel Perspectives on the Global Economic Order". CSIS Report. https://www.csis.org/analysis/parallel-perspectives-global-economic-order.

Gostin, Lawrence O., Eric A. Friedman, and Alexandra Finch. August 4, 2023. "The Global Health Architecture: Governance and International Institutions to Advance Population Health Worldwide". *Milbank Quarterly*. Vol. 101. No. S1: Special Centennial Issue: The Future of Population Health: Challenges & Opportunities, pp. 734–769. https://papers.ssrn.com/sol3/papers.cfm?abstract_id=4434217.

Gouglas, Dimitrios, Mario Christodoulou, Stanley A. Plotkin, and Richard Hatchett. 2019. "CEPI: Driving Progress Toward Epidemic Preparedness and Response". *Epidemiologic Reviews*. Vol. 41, No. 1, p. 28, pp. 28–33.

Government of Japan. 2017. "Be Alert for Old and New Disease, Tuberculosis!". https://www.gcv-online.go.jp/useful/article/201509/3.html.

Granmo, Anders and Pieter Fourie. 2021. *Health Norms and the Governance of Global Development: The Invention of Global Health*. New York: Routledge.

Group of Seven (G7). May 8, 2022. "G7 Leaders' Statement". https://www.mofa.go.jp/mofaj/files/100341354.pdf.

Hamaguchi, Nobuaki and Danielly Ramos, eds. 2022. *Brazil-Japan Cooperation: From Complementarity to Shared Value*. Singapore: Springer.

Harris, Rob. June 23, 2022. "Poliovirus Detected in London Sewage, National Incident Declared". *Sydney Morning Herald*. https://www.smh.com.au/world/europe/polio-virus-detected-in-london-sewage-national-incident-declared-20220623-p5avw2.html.

Hasegawa, Tomoe. April 25, 2020. "Korona Wakuchin, Nihon ga Attoteki ni Deokureru Jijo (Reasons Why Japan Seriously Lags Behind in Developing Coronavirus Vaccines)". https://toyokeizai.net/articles/-/346439?page=4.

Health and Global Policy Institute (HGPI). April 20, 2022. "[Policy Recommendations] Recommendations for the G7 Hiroshima Summit by the C7 Global Health Working Group". https://hgpi.org/en/research/ph-20230420.html.

Health and Global Policy Institute (HGPI). August 22, 2022. "The Public Opinion Survey on Global Health". https://hgpi.org/en/research/gh-survey 202208.html.

Heath, Michael. August 23, 2021. "IMF Urges $650b SDR Injection Be Directed to Covid's Hardest Hit". *Bloomberg*. https://www.bloomberg.com/news/articles/2021-08-23/imf-urges-650b-sdr-injection-be-directed-to-covid-s-hardest-hit.

Hiroshima G7 Global Health Task Force. 2022. "Promote Global Solidarity to Advance Health-System Resilience: Proposals for the G7 Meetings in Japan". *Lancet*. Vol. 401, No. 10385, pp. 1319–1321.

Hiroshima G7 Global Health Task Force, Executive Committee on Global Health and Human Security. 2023. "Promoting Global Solidarity to Advance Health System Resilience: Recommendations for the G7 Meetings in Japan". Japan Center for International Exchange (JCIE). https://www.jcie.org/wp-content/uploads/2023/04/Hiroshima-G7-Global-Health-Task-Force-Recommendations.pdf.

Holmes, David. August 30, 2011. "Keizo Takemi: A Catalytic Charisma". *Lancet*. Vol. 378, No. 9796, p. 1065.

Holmes, David. 2013. "The GHIT Fund Shows Its Cards". *Nature Reviews Drug Discovery*. Vol. 12, p. 894.

Hosoda, Miwako, Hajime Inoue, Yasuo Miyazawa, Eiji Kusumi, and Kenji Shibuya. 2012. "Vaccine-Associated Paralytic Poliomyelitis in Japan". *Lancet*. Vol. 379, No. 9815, p. 520.

Hotez, Peter J. 2020. *Forgotten People Forgotten Diseases: The Neglected Tropical Diseases and Their Impact on Global Health and Development*. Third Edition. Washington, DC: Wiley.

Hutchison, Hayley. 2023. "The Road to UHC: The GFF's Catalytic Role in Supporting PHC Toward the Achievement of UHC". Japan Center for International Exchange (JCIE). https://www.jcie.org/wp-content/uploads/2023/10/JCIE-GFF-PHC-UHC-Report-final.pdf.

IFFIm. July 18, 2019. "IFFIm Issues NOK600 Million Vaccine Bonds". https://iffim.org/press-releases/iffim-issues-nok600-million-vaccine-bonds.

Infectious Disease Surveillance Center. 2012. "Reported Cases of Poliomyelitis in Japan, 1947–1994". https://idsc.niid.go.jp/iasr/18/203/graph/f203-1.gif.

Infectious Disease Surveillance Center. 2000. "Imported Dengue Fever in Japan". *Infectious Agents Surveillance Report*. Vol. 21, No. 6. http://idsc.nih.go.jp/iasr/21/244/tpc244.html.

Ishii, Masato. August 17, 2016. "Hansen's Disease in Japan: The Lingering Legacy of Discrimination". *Nippon.com*. https://www.nippon.com/en/features/c02703/?pnum=1.

Iskra Industry. 2001–2015. "History". http://www.iskra.co.jp/tabid/268/Default.aspx.

Jackson, Alex. June 16, 2022. "Dengue Fever a Growing Threat in Asia". *Japan Times*. https://www.japantimes.co.jp/news/2022/06/16/asia-pacific/science-health-asia-pacific/dengue-fever-asia/.

Jacovella, Diane, Timothy G. Evans, Mariam Claeson, Ruth Kagia, and Ariel Pablos-Mendez. 2016. "Global Financing Facility: Where Will the Funds Come from?" *Lancet*. Vol. 387, No. 10014, pp. 121–122.

Japan Alliance on Global Neglected Tropical Diseases (JAGNTD). 2021. "Japan Alliance on Global Neglected Tropical Disease". https://jagntd.org/.

Japan Center for International Exchange (JCIE). 2009. "G8 Hokkaido Toyako Summit Follow-Up Global Action for Health System Strengthening Policy Recommendations to the G8 (by Task Force on Global Action for Health System Strengthening)". https://www.jcie.org/wp-content/uploads/2021/07/takemi-full.pdf.

Japan Center for International Exchange (JCIE). 2020. "Japan's Global Health Diplomacy in the Post-COVID Era: The Paradigm Shift Needed on ODA and Related Policies: Recommendations". https://www.jcie.org/wp-content/uploads/2020/12/Overview-report-e-122120.pdf.

Japan Center for International Exchange (JCIE). 2021. "Japan's Global Health Diplomacy in the Post-COVID Era: The Paradigm Shift Needed on ODA and Related Policies". https://www.jcie.org/wp-content/uploads/2021/03/Full-DAH-report-final-web.pdf.

Japan Center for International Exchange (JCIE). 2021. "The Global Financing Facility for Women, Children and Adolescents (GFF)". https://www.jcie.or.jp/japan/wp/wp-content/uploads/2020/09/GFF090920.pdf.

Japan Center for International Exchange (JCIE). 2021. "The Global Financing Facility for Women, Children and Adolescents (GFF)". https://www.jcie.or.jp/japan/wp/wp-content/uploads/2021/12/GFF_Nutrition_full_ENG.pdf.

Japan Center for International Exchange (JCIE). January 21, 2021. "Investing in Nutrition: Role of Catalytic Financing". https://www.jcie.or.jp/japan/report/activity-report-14687/.

Japan Center for International Exchange (JCIE). October 2021. "GFF Monitor". No. 3. https://www.jcie.or.jp/japan/wp/wp-content/uploads/2021/10/6b2a5fd37b47ec2ea21099b0dad69a50-1.pdf.

Japan Center for International Exchange (JCIE). 2022. "Hiroshima G7 Global Health Task Force". https://www.jcie.org/programs/global-health-and-human-security/executive-committee-on-global-health-and-human-security/2023-g7-ghtaskforce/.

Japan Center for International Exchange (JCIE). 2022–2023. "Hiroshima G7 Global Health Task Force". https://www.jcie.org/programs/global-health-and-human-security/executive-committee-on-global-health-and-human-security/2023-g7-ghtaskforce/.

Japan Center for International Exchange (JCIE). June 27, 2023. "Hiroshima G7 Global Health Follow-Up Initiative Kick-off Event: Reflections on the 2023 G7". https://www.jcie.org/programs/global-health-and-human-security/executive-committee-on-global-health-and-human-security/2023-g7-ghtaskforce/hiroshima-g7-follow-up-initiative-kickoff/.

Japan Global Health Working Group. 2016. "Protecting Human Security: Proposals for the G7 Ise-Shima Summit in Japan". *Lancet*. Vol. 387, No. 10033, pp. 2155–2162.

Japan Institute for Global Health (JIGH). 2011–2014. "Polio". http://jigh.org/en/activity/project/polio.html.

Japan Institute for Global Health (JIGH). August 4, 2015. "A Resolution to Support Polio Eradication for Children in the World" Submitted to Vice-Foreign Minister Yasuhide Nakayama". http://jigh.org/news/jigh/2390.

Japan International Cooperation Agency (JICA). 2014. "JICA Signs Innovative Financing Agreement with Gates Foundation for Polio Eradication in Nigeria". https://www.jica.go.jp/usa/english/office/others/newsletter/2014/1409_10_02.html.

Japan International Cooperation Agency (JICA). January 2021. "Special Report Revisiting Human Security in Today's Context Security and Dignity for All". https://www.jica.go.jp/english/publications/j-world/2101_03.html.

Japan International Cooperation Agency (JICA). 2022. "About ODA in the World". https://www.jica.go.jp/aboutoda/basic/05.html.

Japan News. September 30, 2021. "Suntory Holdings Limited Suntory Group Global Health Management x Sustainability Initiative 'One Suntory Walk'". https://re-how.net/all/1420090/.

Japan News. August 28, 2022. "Nuclear Disarmament on Kishida's Mind for Hiroshima G7 Summit Next Year". https://japannews.yomiuri.co.jp/politics/politics-government/20220828-54608/.

Japan Times. April 27, 2019. "Improving Health Practices through a Hands-on Approach". https://www.japantimes.co.jp/2019/08/27/special-supplements/improving-health-practices-hands-approach/.

Japan Times. January 12, 2021. "Suga and Gates Say Vaccines for Developing Countries Key for Olympics". https://www.japantimes.co.jp/news/2021/01/12/national/suga-gates-vaccines-developing-countries-olympics/.

Japan Times. January 31, 2021. "Navalny, WHO and Thunberg Among Nominees for Nobel Peace Prize". https://www.japantimes.co.jp/news/2021/01/31/world/nobel-peace-prize-nominees/.

Japan Times. June 3, 2021. "Japan Pledges $800 Million for Global COVID-19 Vaccination Effort". https://www.japantimes.co.jp/news/2021/06/03/national/science-health/japan-covax-donation/.

Japan Times. February 17, 2022. "Japan Stepping Up COVID Vaccine Diplomacy, Without Strings Attached". https://www.japantimes.co.jp/news/2022/02/17/national/japan-covid19-vaccine-diplomacy/.

Japan Times. March 24, 2022. "New Agency Aims to Offer Seamless Support for Children in Japan". https://www.japantimes.co.jp/news/2022/03/24/national/japan-children-agency/.

Japan Times. June 20, 2022. "Japan Seeking to Increase ODA Budget to Support Kishida's Diplomacy Vision". https://www.japantimes.co.jp/news/2022/06/20/national/increase-oda-budget-kishida/.

Japan Times. June 28, 2022. "Japan to Host G7 Summit in Hiroshima Next May". https://www.japantimes.co.jp/news/2022/06/28/national/g7-hiroshima-summit/.

Japan Times. August 26, 2022. "Prospects Bright as Investment Climbs". https://www.japantimes.co.jp/2022/08/26/special-supplements/prospects-bright-investment-climbs/.

Japan Times. August 29, 2022. "Kishida Shows Leadership at TICAD on Global Health and Security". https://www.japantimes.co.jp/opinion/2022/08/29/commentary/japan-commentary/japan-ticad-pledge/.

Jiji. September 4, 2022. "Tojokoku no Iryokaizen wa Nihon no Rieki (Improvement of Medical Care in Developing Countries Is in Japan's Interest)". https://www.jiji.com/jc/v8?id=202209bill-gates-fukabori.

Jones, Marc. April 7, 2009. "ECB's Stark Raps Move to Boost IMF Drawing Rights". *Reuters*. https://jp.reuters.com/article/uk-ecb-stark-sb/ecbs-stark-raps-move-to-boost-imf-drawing-rights-idUKTRE5362AQ20090407/.

Kajimoto, Tetsushi. April 6, 2021. "Japan Backs New IMF Allocation, U.S. Calls for Minimum Corp Tax". *Reuters*. https://www.reuters.com/article/us-g20-debt-japan-idUSKBN2BT08I/.

Kaneda, Yudai, Kenzo Takahashi, Akihiko Ozaki, and Tetsuya Tanimoto. 2023. "Global Vaccine Equity: The G7's Commitment and Challenge". *GHM Open*. Letter, pp. 1–2.

Kantei. 2023. "The Study Group on Impact Investment for Global Health" (Final Report March 2023 Executive Summary). https://www.kantei.go.jp/jp/singi/kenkouiryou/en/pdf/health_final_report.pdf.

Kato, Kazuyo. August 29, 2022. "Kishida Shows Leadership at TICAD on Global Health and Security". *Japan Times*. https://www.japantimes.co.jp/opi nion/2022/08/29/commentary/japan-commentary/japan-ticad-pledge/.

Katow, Shigetaka. 2010. "Polio". *Modern Media*. Vol. 56, No. 3, pp. 61–68. https://www.eiken.co.jp/uploads/modern_media/literature/MM1003_ 03.pdf.

Katsuno, Kei. 2021. "Japan's Innovation for Global Health: GHIT's Catalytic Role". *Parasitology International*. Vol. 80. https://www.sciencedirect.com/ science/article/pii/S1383576920301823?via%3Dihub.

Keath, Lee. November 9, 2021. "Emaciated Children in Kabul Hospital Underscore Rising Hunger in Afghanistan". *The Diplomat*. https://thediplomat. com/2021/11/emaciated-children-in-kabul-hospital-underscore-rising-hun ger-in-afghanistan/.

Keidanren. March 11, 2021. "Exchange Opinions on the Current Situation and the Future Agenda of ODA". http://www.keidanren.or.jp/journal/times/ 2021/0311_05.html.

Kelland, Kate. March 10, 2021. "Coalition Eyes 100-day Target for New Vaccines against Disease Epidemics". *Reuters*. https://www.reuters.com/art icle/us-health-coronavirus-vaccines-cepit-idUSKBN2B201K.

Keller, Janeen Madan, Rachel Silverman, Julia Kaufman, and Amanda Glassman. 2021. "Prioritizing Public Spending on Health in Lower-Income Countries: The Role of the Global Financing Facility for Women, Children and Adolescents". *CGD Policy Paper*. No. 246, pp. 1–48.

Kenzo Fujisue Official Blog. November 19, 2020. "The Diet Task Force on Global Polio Eradication Was Held". https://ameblo.jp/fujisue-kenzo/entry- 12644410496.html.

Kenzo Fujisue Official Blog. October 13, 2022. "Distributing Vaccines to the Children in the World: The Diet Task Force on Global Polio Eradication Was Held". https://ameblo.jp/fujisue-kenzo/entry-12769308034.html.

Kishida, Fumio. January 28, 2023. "Human Security and Universal Health Coverage: Japan's Vision for the G7 Hiroshima Summit". *Lancet*. Vol. 401, No. 10373, pp. 246–247.

Kobayashi, Teruyuki. 2019. "The Control of Lymphatic Filariasis in Japan". *Japanese Journal of History of Pharmacy*. Vol. 54, No. 2, pp. 83–88.

Komeito. October 17, 2020. "Gavi CEO Thanks Komeito for COVAX Support". https://www.komei.or.jp/komeinews/p124659/.

Komeito. June 17, 2021. "Gates Foundation Commends Komeito on COVAX Work". https://www.komei.or.jp/en/news/detail/20210617_28514.

Komeito. December 3, 2021. "Adequate Financial Contributions to International Organizations". https://www.komei.or.jp/komeinews/p218113/.

Komeito. January 14, 2023. "CEPI CEO Calls for Japan, Komeito and G7 to Continue Fight against Infectious Diseases". https://www.komei.or.jp/en/news/detail/20230114_28726.

Komei Shimbun. May 11, 2021. "Wakuchin Kyokyu Kobakkusu (Vaccine Supply through the COVAX Facility)".

Komei Shimbun. February 17, 2022. "CEPI e Shikin Kyoshutsu ga Hitsuyo (Financial Support for CEPI Is Necessary)".

Komori, Yoshihisa. November 8, 2018. "Japan's ODA to China: End of a Momentous Foreign Policy Failure". *Japan Forward*. https://japan-forward.com/japans-oda-to-china-end-of-a-momentous-foreign-policy-failure/.

Kumai, Hiromi. June 26, 2020. "Routine Vaccination Rate of Three-Year-Old Children Decreased". *Asahi Shimbun*. https://www.asahi.com/articles/ASN6T5JMFN6LULBJ01X.html.

Kunii, Osamu. 2019. *Sekai Saikyo Soshiki no Tsukurikata: Kansensho to Tatakau Global Fund no Chosen (How to Create the World's Strongest Organization: Challenge by the Global Fund to Fight Infectious Diseases)*. Tokyo: Chikuma Shobo.

Kyodo News. April 8, 2022. "Japan PM Pledges $500 Mil. for Global Vaccine-sharing Efforts". https://english.kyodonews.net/news/2022/04/7e83ee83ccab-japan-pm-pledges-500-mil-to-global-far-vaccine-sharing-efforts.html.

Lehman, Howard. 2005. "Japan's Foreign Aid Policy to Africa Since the Tokyo International Conference on African Development". *Pacific Affairs*. Vol. 78, No. 3, pp. 423–442.

Lawler, Daniel. December 23, 2022. "Three Years into COVID-19: Are We Ready for the Next Pandemic?" *Japan Times*. https://www.japantimes.co.jp/news/2022/12/23/asia-pacific/three-years-covid-19-pandemic/.

Lindgren, Wrenn Yennie. 2020. "WIN-WIN! with ODA-man: Legitimizing Development Assistance Policy in Japan". *Pacific Review*. Vol. 34, No. 4, pp. 633–663.

Mainichi Shimbun November 27, 2017. "Japan Needs Long-Term Plan to Tackle Vicious Poverty Cycle". https://mainichi.jp/english/articles/20171127/p2a/00m/0na/016000c.

Mainichi. December 24, 2021. "Grant Aid ODA to Be Slightly Increased by LDP's Support, Outnegotiating the Finance Ministry". https://mainichi.jp/articles/20211224/k00/00m/010/273000c.

Malaria No More Japan. March 26, 2021. "Welcome to the Establishment of the Parliamentary Group to End Malaria by 2030 in Japan". https://malarianomore.jp/wp_core/wp-content/uploads/2021/03/Parliamentary-Group-Launch_pressrelease_0326_final.pdf.

Malaria No More Japan. July 19, 2022. "Request for Malaria Control along with the Promotion of Irrigated Rice Cultivation in Sub-Saharan Africa". https://malarianomore.jp/wp_core/wp-content/uploads/2022/07/20220719policyrecommendation_Eng.pdf.

Martin, Eric. August 19, 2021. "IMF Curbs Afghanistan's Funding Access, Squeezing Taliban". *Bloomberg*. https://www.bloomberg.com/news/articles/2021-08-18/imf-says-afghanistan-can-t-access-sdrs-or-fund-s-resources.

McAdams, David, Kaci Kennedy McDade, Osondu Ogbuoji, Matthew Johnson, Siddharth Dixit, and Gavin Yamey. 2020. "Incentivising Wealthy Nations to Participate in the COVID-19 Vaccine Global Access Facility (COVAX): A Game Theory Perspective". *BMJ Global Health*. Vol. 5, No. 11, pp. 1–7.

McInnes, Colin and Kelly Lee. 2012. *Global Health and International Relations*. Cambridge: Polity Press.

McInnes, Colin, Kelley Lee, and Jeremy Youde, eds. 2020. *The Oxford Handbook of Global Health Politics*. Oxford: Oxford University Press.

Ministry of Finance. October 14, 2021. "Statement by the Honorable SUZUKI Shunichi Governor of the IMF for Japan at the Forty-Fourth Meeting of the International Monetary and Financial Committee". https://www.mof.go.jp/english/policy/international_policy/imf/imfc/imfc_20211014_2.pdf.

Ministry of Finance Japan. 2022. "Sokatsu Chosahyo: The Global Fund (Summary Survey on the Global Fund)". https://www.mof.go.jp/policy/budget/topics/budget_execution_audit/fy2022/sy0407/7.pdf.

Ministry of Finance Japan. April 12, 2023. "Japan's Statement at the 107th Meeting of the Development Committee (Joint Ministerial Committee of the Boards of Governors of the Bank and the Fund) (Washington, DC–April 12, 2023)". https://www.mof.go.jp/english/policy/international_policy/imf/dc/20230412_2.html.

Ministry of Foreign Affairs of Japan. 1993. "List of the Participating Delegations of the Tokyo International Conference on African Development (October 5–6, 1993, Tokyo, Japan)". https://www.mofa.go.jp/region/africa/ticad/list/index.html.

Ministry of Foreign Affairs of Japan. October 5, 1993. "Keynote Speech by Prime Minister Morihiro Hosokawa in TICAD". https://www.mofa.go.jp/mofaj/press/enzetsu/05/eos_1005.html.

Ministry of Foreign Affairs of Japan. October 6, 1993. "The Tokyo Declaration on African Development". https://www.mofa.go.jp/mofaj/area/ticad/tc_senge.html.

Ministry of Foreign Affairs of Japan. 1997. "Japan's ODA Charter". https://www.mofa.go.jp/policy/oda/summary/1997/09.html.

Ministry of Foreign Affairs of Japan. 1998. "The Tokyo Declaration on African Development in TICAD 2". https://www.mofa.go.jp/mofaj/area/ticad/kodo_1.html#4-1-2.

Ministry of Foreign Affairs of Japan. October 19, 1998. "Keynote Speech by Prime Minister Keizo Obuchi in TICAD 2". https://www.mofa.go.jp/mofaj/press/enzetsu/10/eos_1019.html.

Ministry of Foreign Affairs of Japan. October 19–20, 1998. "Tokyo International Conference on African Development Tokyo, October 19th-21st, 1998 List of Participants". https://www.mofa.go.jp/region/africa/ticad2/list/index.html.

Ministry of Foreign Affairs of Japan. October 21, 1998. "Japan's New Africa Support Program based on Action Plan in TICAD 2". https://www.mofa.go.jp/mofaj/area/ticad/tc_progr.html.

Ministry of Foreign Affairs of Japan. July 21–23, 2000. "Kyushu-Okinawa Summit". https://www.mofa.go.jp/policy/economy/summit/2000/index.html.

Ministry of Foreign Affairs of Japan. July 23, 2000. "G8 Communique Okinawa 2000". https://www.mofa.go.jp/policy/economy/summit/2000/documents/communique.html.

Ministry of Foreign Affairs of Japan. 2003. "Highlights of the Summary by the Chair of TICAD III". https://www.mofa.go.jp/region/africa/ticad3/chair-2.html.

Ministry of Foreign Affairs of Japan. September 29, 2003. "Opening Remarks by Mr. Yoshiro Mori, Chairperson of TICAD III". https://www.mofa.go.jp/region/africa/ticad3/opening.html.

Ministry of Foreign Affairs of Japan. September 29, 2003. "Keynote Speech by Prime Minister Junichiro Koizumi at the Third Tokyo International Conference on African Development (TICAD III)". https://www.mofa.go.jp/region/africa/ticad3/pmspeech.html.

Ministry of Foreign Affairs of Japan. June 30, 2005. "Prime Minister Koizumi Pledges 'US$ 500 Million for the Coming Years' to the Global Fund, Reiterates US$ 5 Billion Pledge over 5 Years for Health in ODA". https://www.mofa.go.jp/announce/announce/2005/6/0630.html.

Ministry of Foreign Affairs of Japan. June 30, 2005. "Address by Prime Minister Junichiro Koizumi at the Commemorative Symposium on the Fifth Anniversary of the Kyusyu-Okinawa Summit: East Asian Regional Response to HIV/AIDS, Tuberculosis and Malaria". https://www.mofa.go.jp/policy/health_c/gfatm/address0506.html.

Ministry of Foreign Affairs of Japan. May 23, 2008. "Opening Remarks by H.E. Mr. Yasuo Fukuda, Prime Minister of Japan on the Occasion of "From Okinawa to Toyako: Dealing with Communicable Diseases as Global Human Security Threats". https://www.mofa.go.jp/policy/health_c/remark0805.html.

Ministry of Foreign Affairs of Japan. May 28, 2008. "Address by H.E. Mr. Yasuo Fukuda, Prime Minister of Japan at the Opening Session of the Fourth Tokyo

International Conference on African Development (TICAD IV)". https://www.mofa.go.jp/region/africa/ticad/ticad4/pm/address.html.

Ministry of Foreign Affairs of Japan. 2008. "G8 Hokkaido-Toyako Summit". https://www.mofa.go.jp/policy/economy/summit/2008/index.html.

Ministry of Foreign Affairs of Japan. May 23, 2008. "Opening Remarks by H.E. Mr. Yasuo Fukuda, Prime Minister of Japan on the Occasion of 'From Okinawa to Toyako: Dealing with Communicable Diseases as Global Human Security Threats'". https://www.mofa.go.jp/policy/health_c/remark0805.html.

Ministry of Foreign Affairs of Japan. May 28–30, 2008a. "The Fourth Tokyo International Conference on African Development (TICAD IV) in Yokohama 28–30 May, 2008". https://www.mofa.go.jp/region/africa/ticad/ticad4/index.html.

Ministry of Foreign Affairs of Japan. May 28–30, 2008b. "Towards a Vibrant Africa a Continent of Hope and Opportunity". https://www.mofa.go.jp/region/africa/ticad/ticad4/initiative.pdf.

Ministry of Foreign Affairs of Japan. July 2008. "Toyako Framework Action for Global Health". https://www.mofa.go.jp/policy/economy/summit/2008/doc/pdf/20080728_02.pdf.

Ministry of Foreign Affairs of Japan. July 8, 2008. "Toyako Framework for Action on Global Health: Report of the G8 Health Experts Group". https://www.mofa.go.jp/policy/economy/summit/2008/doc/pdf/0708_09_en.pdf.

Ministry of Foreign Affairs of Japan. October 5, 2010. "Speech by State Secretary for Foreign Affairs Yutaka BANNO at the Third Voluntary Replenishment Conference of the Global Fund to Fight AIDS, Tuberculosis and Malaria". https://www.mofa.go.jp/announce/svm/speech101006.html.

Ministry of Foreign Affairs of Japan. 2011. "Japan's Official Development Assistance White Paper 2011". https://www.mofa.go.jp/policy/oda/white/2011/html/keyword/keyword02.html.

Ministry of Foreign Affairs of Japan. 2013. "Japan's Official Development Assistance Charter". https://www.mofa.go.jp/policy/oda/reform/revision0308.pdf.

Ministry of Foreign Affairs of Japan. March 11, 2013. "Exchange of Notes Signing Ceremony for the Grant Aid Project for the Project for the Control and Eradication of Poliomyelitis". https://www.mofa.go.jp/mofaj/press/release/25/3/0311_06.html.

Ministry of Foreign Affairs of Japan. March 12, 2013. "Courtesy Call on Vice-Foreign Minister Masaji Matsuyama by Mr. Mark Dybul, Executive Director of the Global Fund". https://www.mofa.go.jp/mofaj/annai/honsho/fuku/matsuyama/wf_130312.html.

Ministry of Foreign Affairs of Japan. March 14, 2013. "Review of Japan's Official Development Assistance Charter". https://www.mofa.go.jp/policy/oda/reform/review0303.html.

Ministry of Foreign Affairs of Japan. June 1, 2013. "The Africa that Joins in Partnership with Japan Is Brighter Still: Address by H.E. Mr. Shinzo Abe, Prime Minister of Japan, at the Opening Session of the Fifth Tokyo International Conference on African Development (TICAD V)". https://www.mofa.go.jp/files/000005500.pdf.

Ministry of Foreign Affairs of Japan. June 3, 2013. "Fifth Tokyo International Conference on African Development (TICAD V)". https://www.mofa.go.jp/region/page6e_000075.html, https://www.mofa.go.jp/region/page2e_000002.html.

Ministry of Foreign Affairs of Japan. June 3, 2013. "Yokohama Declaration 2013: Hand in Hand with a More Dynamic Africa". https://www.mofa.go.jp/region/page3e_000053.html.

Ministry of Foreign Affairs of Japan. December 3, 2013. "Speech by Parliamentary Vice-Minister for Foreign Affairs Seiji KIHARA at the Fourth Voluntary Replenishment Conference of the Global Fund to Fight AIDS, Tuberculosis and Malaria". https://www.mofa.go.jp/mofaj/files/000023126.pdf.

Ministry of Foreign Affairs of Japan. March 7, 2014. "Exchange of Notes Signing Ceremony for the Grant Aid Project for the Project for the Control and Eradication of Poliomyelitis". https://www.mofa.go.jp/mofaj/press/release/press4_000698.html.

Ministry of Foreign Affairs of Japan. 2015. "Decision on Development Cooperation Charter". https://www.mofa.go.jp/files/000067702.pdf.

Ministry of Foreign Affairs of Japan. January 21, 2015. "Exchange of Notes on Grant Aid to the 'Project for Infectious Diseases Prevention for Children' in Afghanistan through the UNICEF". https://www.mofa.go.jp/mofaj/press/release/press4_001678.html.

Ministry of Foreign Affairs of Japan. February 10, 2015. "Cabinet Decision on the Development Cooperation Charter". https://www.mofa.go.jp/mofaj/gaiko/oda/files/000067701.pdf.

Ministry of Foreign Affairs of Japan. March 8, 2015. "Rebuttal Statement against the Editorial of *Japan Times*: 'Aid That Could Foment Conflict' (February 20, 2015)". https://www.mofa.go.jp/policy/oda/page_000139.html.

Ministry of Foreign Affairs of Japan. December 17, 2015. "Remarks by Foreign Minister Kishida at the 5th Replenishment Preparatory Meeting of the Global Fund (17 December, 2015 at Tokyo Prince Hotel)". https://www.mofa.go.jp/ic/ghp/page24e_000124.html.

Ministry of Foreign Affairs of Japan. 2016. "G7 Ise-Shima Vision for Global Health". https://www.mofa.go.jp/files/000160273.pdf.

Ministry of Foreign Affairs of Japan. May 26–27, 2016. "G7 Ise-Shima Leaders' Declaration G7 Ise-Shima Summit, 26–27 May 2016". https://www.mofa.go.jp/files/000160266.pdf.

Ministry of Foreign Affairs of Japan. May 27, 2016. "G7 Ise-Shima Summit". https://www.mofa.go.jp/ecm/ec/page4e_000457.html.

Ministry of Foreign Affairs of Japan. August 26, 2016. "TICAD VI Nairobi Declaration: Advancing Africa's Sustainable Development Agenda TICAD Partnership for Prosperity". https://www.mofa.go.jp/af/afl/page3e_000 543.html.

Ministry of Foreign Affairs of Japan. August 27, 2016. "Address by Prime Minister Shinzo Abe at the Opening Session of the Sixth Tokyo International Conference on African Development (TICAD VI)". https://www.mofa.go.jp/afr/af2/page4e_000496.html.

Ministry of Foreign Affairs of Japan. August 28, 2016. "Sixth Tokyo International Conference on African Development (TICAD VI)". https://www.mofa.go.jp/af/afl/page3e_000551.html.

Ministry of Foreign Affairs of Japan. October 9–10, 2016. "Speech by State Minister for Foreign Affairs of Japan, Mr. SUZUKI Keisuke". https://www.mofa.go.jp/mofaj/files/000526525.pdf.

Ministry of Foreign Affairs of Japan. June 22, 1997. "Record on Press Conference by Prime Minister Ryutaro Hashimoto in Denver". https://www.mofa.go.jp/mofaj/gaiko/summit/denver/kaiken.html.

Ministry of Foreign Affairs of Japan. May 15–17, 1998. "G8 Birmingham Summit Communiqué". https://www.mofa.go.jp/mofaj/gaiko/summit/birmin98/commun.html.

Ministry of Foreign Affairs of Japan. 2019. "The ABE Initiative-Pilots of African Business". https://www.mofa.go.jp/files/000469595.pdf.

Ministry of Foreign Affairs of Japan. August 28, 2019. "Keynote Address by Mr. Shinzo Abe, Prime Minister of Japan at the Opening Session of the Seventh Tokyo International Conference on African Development (TICAD 7)". https://www.mofa.go.jp/af/afl/page4e_001069.html.

Ministry of Foreign Affairs of Japan. August 28–30, 2019. "The Seventh Tokyo International Conference on African Development (TICAD 7)". https://www.mofa.go.jp/region/africa/ticad/ticad7/index.html.

Ministry of Foreign Affairs of Japan. August 30, 2019. "Yokohama Declaration 2019 Advancing Africa's Development through People, Technology and Innovation". https://www.mofa.go.jp/region/africa/ticad/ticad7/pdf/yokohama_declaration_en.pdf.

Ministry of Foreign Affairs of Japan. March 30, 2020. "Telephone Talk between Prime Minister ABE Shinzo and WHO Director-General Dr. Tedros Adhanom". https://www.mofa.go.jp/page1e_000277.html.

Ministry of Foreign Affairs of Japan. 2021. "Opening Speech by Prime Minister, Mr. Kishida at the Tokyo Nutrition for Growth (N4G) Summit 2021". https://www.mofa.go.jp/files/100269401.pdf.

Ministry of Foreign Affairs of Japan. January 12, 2021. "Telephone Talk between Prime Minister SUGA Yoshihide and Co-Chair of the Bill & Melinda Gates Foundation Bill Gates". https://www.mofa.go.jp/ic/ghp/page4e_001109.html.

Ministry of Foreign Affairs of Japan. 2022. "Gavi COVAX AMC Summit 2022 Statement by H.E. Fumio Kishida, Prime Minister of Japan". https://www.mofa.go.jp/files/100329713.pdf.

Ministry of Foreign Affairs of Japan. 2022. "G7 Hiroshima Vision for Equitable Access to Medical Countermeasure". https://www.mofa.go.jp/files/100506811.pdf.

Ministry of Foreign Affairs of Japan. February 8, 2022. "The Eighth Tokyo International Conference on African Development (TICAD 8) (Tunisia)". https://www.mofa.go.jp/afr/af2/page24e_000325.html.

Ministry of Foreign Affairs of Japan. February 24, 2022. "Courtesy Call on Vice-Foreign Minister Takako Suzuki by Mr. Osamu Kunii as a Management Executive Committee Member of the Global Fund". https://www.mofa.go.jp/mofaj/ic/ghp/page1_001102.html.

Ministry of Foreign Affairs of Japan. April 9, 2022. "Meeting between Akahori Takeshi, Ambassador, Director-General for Global Issues of the Foreign Ministry and Mr. Peter Sands, Executive Director of the Global Fund". https://www.mofa.go.jp/mofaj/press/release/press1_000824.html.

Ministry of Foreign Affairs of Japan. April 12, 2022. "Vaccine Donation to Cambodia by Japan-Australia-India-U.S. (Quad)". https://www.mofa.go.jp/press/release/press1e_000283.html.

Ministry of Foreign Affairs of Japan. April 21, 2022. "Courtesy Call on Foreign Minister Hayashi Yoshimasa by Mr. Peter Sands, Executive Director of the Global Fund". https://www.mofa.go.jp/press/release/press1e_000285.html.

Ministry of Foreign Affairs of Japan. May 2022. "Japan's COVID-19 Vaccine-Related Support". https://www.mofa.go.jp/files/100226669.pdf.

Ministry of Foreign Affairs of Japan. August 4, 2022. "Results Overview of the Tokyo Nutrition for Growth (N4G) Summit 2021 (Day 1: High Level Sessions)". https://www.mofa.go.jp/ic/ghp/page6e_000264.html.

Ministry of Foreign Affairs of Japan. August 27, 2022. "Eighth Tokyo International Conference on African Development (TICAD 8) (Day 1: Opening Session and Plenary 1)". https://www.mofa.go.jp/afr/af2/page1e_000469.html.

Ministry of Foreign Affairs of Japan. December 16, 2022. "National Security Strategy of Japan" (provisional translation), p. 17. https://www.cas.go.jp/jp/siryou/221216anzenhoshou/nss-e.pdf.

Ministry of Foreign Affairs of Japan. May 20, 2023. "G7 Hiroshima Leaders' Communiqué". https://www.mofa.go.jp/files/100506907.pdf.

Ministry of Foreign Affairs of Japan. August 8, 2023. "Decision on the Host City of Ninth Tokyo International Conference on African Development (TICAD 9)". https://www.mofa.go.jp/press/release/press7e_000026.html.

Ministry of Foreign Affairs of Japan. October 10, 2023. "Development Cooperation Charter: Japan's Contributions to the Sustainable Development of a Free and Open World". https://www.mofa.go.jp/mofaj/gaiko/oda/files/100514705.pdf.

Ministry of Health, Labour and Welfare of Japan. 2016. "IPV Vaccination Schedule in Other Countries". https://www.mhlw.go.jp/file/05-Shingikai-10601000-Daijinkanboukouseikagakuka-Kouseikagakuka/0000145361.pdf.

Ministry of Health, Labour and Welfare of Japan. 2016. "Fifth Dose of IPV". https://www.mhlw.go.jp/file/05-Shingikai-10601000-Daijinkanboukouseikagakuka-Kouseikagakuka/0000145358.pdf.

Ministry of Health, Labour and Welfare of Japan. January 29, 2018. "Basic Information on Polio and Polio Vaccines". https://www.mhlw.go.jp/bunya/kenkou/polio/qa.html.

Ministry of Health, Labour and Welfare of Japan. 2020. "Annual Report on the Registered Number of Tuberculosis Infection". https://www.mhlw.go.jp/stf/seisakunitsuite/bunya/0000175095_00004.html.

Ministry of Health, Labour and Welfare of Japan. September 15, 2020. "Overview of Press Interview by Minister Kato". https://www.mhlw.go.jp/stf/kaiken/daijin/0000194708_00276.html.

Ministry of Health, Labour and Welfare of Japan. June 4, 2021. "International Cooperation through Domestically Produced Coronavirus Vaccines". https://www.mhlw.go.jp/stf/newpage_19070.html.

Ministry of Health, Labour and Welfare. February 25, 2022. "Nihon kara Sepi ni Taisuru Aratana Kyoshutsu ni tsuite (Japan's Pledge on Additional Donation to CEPI)". https://www.mhlw.go.jp/stf/newpage_24098.html.

Ministry of Health, Labour and Welfare of Japan. May 13–14, 2023. "G7 Health Ministers' Meeting in Nagasaki". https://www.mhlw.go.jp/stf/seisakunitsuite/bunya/hokabunya/kokusai/g8/g7health2023_en.html.

Ministry of Health, Labour and Welfare of Japan. May 13–14, 2023. "G7 Nagasaki Health Ministers' Communiqué". https://www.mhlw.go.jp/content/10500000/001098603.pdf.

Ministry of Health, Labour and Welfare of Japan. May 13–14, 2023. "G7 Global Plan for UHC Action Agenda". https://www.mhlw.go.jp/content/10500000/001098604.pdf.

Mitsubishi UFJ Research and Consulting. 2021. "Global Health Business Leader Coalition Handed out a Request Form to PM Suga". https://www.digita lsociety.murc.jp/globalhealth/architecture/policy/20210427_coalition_en/ index.html.

miup. 2022. "About Us". https://miup.jp/aboutus/.

Miyoshi, Masahiro, Shima Yoshizumi, Masaru Jinushi, Setsuko Ishida, Toyo Okui, Motohiko Okano, Masayo Shouji, Sanae Tanaka, Junichi Saigusa, Akihisa Mori, Hiroki Tanabe, Ryo Yamaguchi, Yorihiro Nishimura, and Hiroyuki Shimizu. 2010. "A Case of Paralytic Poliomyelitis Associated with Poliovirus Vaccine Strains in Hokkaido, Japan". *Japanese Journal of Infectious Diseases*. Vol. 63, No. 3, pp. 216–217.

Mizuho Information & Research Institute. 2017. "Evaluation of Japan's ODA to Africa Through the TICAD Process for the Past 10 Years". https://www. mofa.go.jp/policy/oda/evaluation/FY2017/pdfs/ticad.pdf.

Molyneux, David H., Anarfi Asamoa-Bah, Alan Fenwick, Lorenzo Savioli, and Peter Hotez. 2021. "The History of the Neglected Tropical Disease Movement". *Tropical Medicine and Hygiene*. Vol. 115, No. 2, pp. 169–175.

Mori, Yoshiro. June 5, 2000. "Address by Prime Minister Yoshiro Mori at the Discussion Group on the Kyushu-Okinawa Summit, Okinawa Summit". *"The World and Japan" Database*. https://worldjpn.grips.ac.jp/documents/texts/ summit/20000605.S1E.html.

Morrison, J. Stephen. August 31, 2023. "Dr. Scott Dowell, the Bill & Melinda Gates Foundation: 'I Am Optimistic'". Center for Strategic & International Studies (CSIS). https://www.csis.org/podcasts/commonhealth/dr-scott-dowell-bill-melinda-gates-foundation-i-am-optimistic.

MUFJ Research and Consulting. 2023. "Center on Global Health Architecture". https://www.globalhealth.murc.jp/globalhealth/architecture/index.html.

Nagasaki University. 2022. "The Institute of Tropical Medicine". https://www. tm.nagasaki-u.ac.jp/nekken/en/.

Nagatani, Shiori, Tomoko Yoshida, and Tomoko Suzuki. 2021. "Toward Achieving the SDGs: The GFF's Impact and Challenges and Its Significance for Japan". Japan Center for International Exchange (JCIE). https://www. jcie.org/wp-content/uploads/2021/07/GFF-report-2021-EN-070721_1. pdf.

Nakano, Takashi. 2011. "Japanese Vaccinations and Practices, with Particular Attention to Polio and Pertussis". *Travel Medicine and Infectious Disease*. Vol. 9, No. 4, pp. 169–175.

National Diet Library. March 8, 2011. "Proceedings of the 177 Diet Session. The Committee on Health, Labour and Welfare, the House of Representatives". https://kokkai.ndl.go.jp/#/detail?minId=117704260 X00320110308&spkNum=86&current=9.

National Diet Library. May 18, 2011. "Proceedings of the 177th Diet Session. The Committee on Audit, the House of Councillors". https://kokkai.ndl.go. jp/txt/117714103X00620110518/195 and https://kokkai.ndl.go.jp/txt/ 117714103X00620110518/196.

National Diet Library. March 23, 2016. "Proceedings of the 190th Diet Session. Committee on Health, Labour and Welfare, the House of Councillors". https://kokkai.ndl.go.jp/txt/119014260X00820160323/23 and https:// kokkai.ndl.go.jp/txt/119014260X00820160323/24.

National Diet Library. April 21, 2016. "Proceedings of the 190th Diet Session. Committee on Health, Labour and Welfare, the House of Councillors". https://kokkai.ndl.go.jp/txt/119014260X01520160421/138.

National Diet Library. March 21, 2017. "Proceedings of the 193rd Diet Session. Special Committee on Official Development Assistance, etc., the House of Councillors". https://kokkai.ndl.go.jp/#/detail?minId=119314 580X00220170321&spkNum=26&current=2.

National Diet Library. March 21, 2017. "Proceedings of the 193rd Diet Session. Special Committee on Official Development Assistance, etc., the House of Councillors". https://kokkai.ndl.go.jp/#/detail?minId=119314 580X00220170321&spkNum=27&current=1.

National Diet Library. March 12, 2019. "Proceedings of the 198th Diet Session, Committee on Foreign Affairs and Defense, the House of Councillors". https://kokkai.ndl.go.jp/txt/119813950X00320190312/7.

National Diet Library. August 20, 2020. "Proceedings of the 201st Diet Session. Committee on Health, Labour and Welfare, the House of Councillors". https://kokkai.ndl.go.jp/#/detail?minId=120114260X00220 200820&spkNum=16&current=78.

National Diet Library. October 8, 2020. "Proceedings of the 202nd Diet Session. Cabinet Committee, the House of Councillors". https://kokkai.ndl. go.jp/#/detail?minId=120214889X00120201008&spkNum=97&single and https://kokkai.ndl.go.jp/#/detail?minId=120214889X00120201008&spk Num=98&single.

National Diet Library. November 2, 2020. "Proceedings of the 202nd Diet Session. Budget Committee, the House of Representatives". https://kokkai. ndl.go.jp/#/detail?minId=120305261X00220201102&spkNum=128&single and https://kokkai.ndl.go.jp/txt/120305261X00220201102/129.

National Diet Library. June 11, 2021. "Proceedings of the 204th Diet Session. Committee on Health, Labour and Welfare, the House of Representatives". https://kokkai.ndl.go.jp/#/detail?minId=120404260X02 720210611&spkNum=158&current=30.

National Diet Library. March 23, 2022. "Proceedings of the 208th Diet Session. Special Committee on the Official Development Assistance, etc. and Okinawa and Northern Territories, the House of Councillors". https://kokkai.ndl.go.jp/#/detail?minId=120815359X00420220323&spkNum=56&current=15.

National Diet Library. May 20, 2022. "Proceedings of the 208th Diet Session. Health, Labour and Welfare Committee, the House of Representatives". https://kokkai.ndl.go.jp/#/detail?minId=120804260X02120220520&spkNum=154&current=8.

National Diet Library. October 13, 2022. "Proceeding of the 210th Diet Session. Foreign Affairs Committee, the House of Representatives". https://kokkai.ndl.go.jp/#/detail?minId=121005365X00120221013&spkNum=108&current=5.

National Diet Library. November 24, 2022. "Proceedings of the 210th Diet Session, the Committee on Health, Labour and Welfare, the House of Councillors". https://kokkai.ndl.go.jp/txt/121014260X00820221124/27 and https://kokkai.ndl.go.jp/txt/121014260X00820221124/28.

National Diet Library. March 16, 2023. "Proceeding of the 211th Diet Session. Special Committee on the Official Development Assistance etc. and Okinawa and Northern Territories, the House of Councillors". https://kokkai.ndl.go.jp/#/detail?minId=121115359X00320230316&spkNum=78&current=1.

National Institute of Infectious Diseases. 2017. *IASR*. Vol. 38, No. 3 (No. 445), March 2017, p. 67–68. https://www.niid.go.jp/niid/ja/vaccine-j/1685-idsc/iasr-out/7146-445f01.html.

National Institute of Infectious Diseases. 2018. "Acquired Immunodeficiency Syndrome, AIDS". https://www.niid.go.jp/niid/ja/kansennohanashi/400-aids-intro.html.

Nature Medicine. 2013. "Straight Talk with...BT Slingsby". Vol. 19, No. 1553. https://www.nature.com/articles/nm1213-1553.

NEC. June 6, 2019. "Gavi, NEC, and Simprints to Deploy World's First Scalable Child Fingerprint Identification Solution to Boost Immunization in Developing Countries". https://www.nec.com/en/press/201906/global_20190606_01.html.

NEC. 2022. "AI Technology Is Revolutionizing the Vaccine Development Industry". https://www.nec.com/en/global/sdgs/innovators/nvw2022/report.html.

NEC. Aril 8, 2022. "CEPI Partners with Japan's NEC Group to Develop Artificial Intelligence-designed Broadly Protective Betacoronavirus Vaccine". https://www.nec.com/en/press/202204/global_20220408_02.html.

Nen, Satomi. September 7, 2022. "Japan to Review ODA Policy to Strengthen Indo-Pacific Ties". *Asahi Shimbun*. https://www.asahi.com/ajw/articles/14713027.

NHK World Japan. June 7, 2022. "Kishida's 'New Capitalism' Shifts Emphasis to Growth". https://www3.nhk.or.jp/nhkworld/en/news/videos/20220607211259765/.

NHK. January 14, 2023. "Tech Firm Crunches Data for Next-gen Vaccine". https://www3.nhk.or.jp/nhkworld/en/news/backstories/2181/.

Nikkei Asia. November 30, 2021. "Shionogi and Daiichi Sankyo Join Hunt for Omicron Vaccine". https://asia.nikkei.com/Spotlight/Coronavirus/COVID-vaccines/Shionogi-and-Daiichi-Sankyo-join-hunt-for-omicron-vaccine.

Nikkei Shimbun. August 21, 2021. "Japan's ODA, Highest Record in Its History". https://www.nikkei.com/article/DGKKZO74392650R00C21A8PE8000/.

Nikkei Shimbun. October 22, 2022. "100 Nichi de Wakuchin Sesshu Kyokyu Mezase (Let's Prepare for Vaccine Supply in the 100 Days)". https://www.nikkei.com/article/DGXZQOCB133940T11C22A0000000/.

Nippon.com. November 6, 2018. "After 40 Years, Japan Stops Aid to China". https://www.nippon.com/en/features/h00321/.

Nippon Foundation. 2015. "Addressing Child Poverty". https://www.nippon-foundation.or.jp/en/what/projects/ending_child_poverty.

Nishida, Ippeita. August 10, 2022. "Revising the Development Cooperation Charter: Issues in Linking ODA and Security". Sasakawa Peace Foundation: International Information Network Analysis. https://www.spf.org/iina/en/articles/nishida_02.html.

Nomura, Shuhei, Lisa Yamasaki, Kazuki Shimizu, Cyrus Ghaznavi, and Haruka Sakamoto. 2022. "Japan's Development Assistance for Health: Historical Trends and Prospects for a New Era". *Lancet*. Vol. 22, No. 100403, pp. 1–9.

Okada, Minoru. 2014. *Bokura no Mura kara Polio ga Kieta: Chugoku Santoshohatsu "Kagakuteki Genjitsushugi" no Kokusai Kyoryoku (Poliovirus Disappeared from Our Village: International Cooperation of "Scientific Realism" in Shandong Province of China)*. Tokyo: Saiki Communications.

Osaka Institute of Public Health. April 19, 2021. "April 25 is Malaria Day". http://www.iph.osaka.jp/li/070/20210419160926.html.

Otake, Tomoko. December 12, 2017. "Tokyo-Based Fund CEO Leads Public-private Fight Against Diseases Around Globe". *Japan Times*. https://www.japantimes.co.jp/news/2017/12/12/national/science-health/tokyo-based-fund-ceo-leads-public-private-fight-diseases-around-globe/.

Panda, Ankit. February 9, 2015. "Japan to Open Military Aid Channel". *The Diplomat*. https://thediplomat.com/2015/02/japan-to-open-military-aid-channel/.

Paton, James. September 29, 2021. "Deaths of Women and Children Show Wider Impact of Pandemic". *Bloomberg*. https://www.bloomberg.com/news/articles/2021-09-29/deaths-of-women-and-children-show-wider-impact-of-pandemic#xj4y7vzkg.

PR Times. April 22, 2022. "Japanese Business Leaders' Coalition for Global Health Requested Prime Minister Kishida to Strengthen Japan's

Global Health Activities". https://prtimes.jp/main/html/rd/p/000000009. 000076537.html.

PR Times. August 25, 2022. "Global Health Action Japan 2022". https://prt imes.jp/main/html/rd/p/000000010.000076537.html.

PR Times. December 9, 2022. "The First Global Health Academy". https://prt imes.jp/main/html/rd/p/000000013.000076537.html.

PR Times. March 31, 2023. "The Second Global Health Academy". https://prt imes.jp/main/html/rd/p/000000015.000076537.html.

PR Times. April 24, 2023. "The Third Global Health Academy". https://prt imes.jp/main/html/rd/p/000000016.000076537.html.

PR Times. September 8, 2023. "The Fourth Global Health Academy". https:// prtimes.jp/main/html/rd/p/000000017.000076537.html.

PR Times. November 22, 2023. "The Fifth Global Health Academy". https:// prtimes.jp/main/html/rd/p/000000018.000076537.html.

Prime Minister of Japan and His Cabinet. November 8, 2021. "Outline of Emergency Proposal Toward the Launch of a 'New Form of Capitalism' that Carves Out the Future". https://japan.kantei.go.jp/ongoingtopics/_00001.html.

Prime Minister of Japan and His Cabinet. 2022. "Global Health Strategy Outline". https://www.kantei.go.jp/jp/singi/kenkouiryou/en/pdf/final_ GHS_outline.pdf

Prime Minister of Japan and His Cabinet. April 23, 2022. "Speech by Prime Minister KISHIDA Fumio at the 4th Asia-Pacific Water Summit". https:// japan.kantei.go.jp/101_kishida/statement/202204/_00017.html.

Prime Minister of Japan and His Cabinet. May 24, 2022. "Global Health Strategy of Japan". https://www.kantei.go.jp/jp/singi/kenkouiryou/en/ pdf/final_GHS.pdf.

Prime Minister of Japan and His Cabinet. August 27, 2022. "Opening Speech by Prime Minister KISHIDA Fumio at the Opening Session of the Eighth Tokyo International Conference on African Development (TICAD 8)". https:// japan.kantei.go.jp/101_kishida/statement/202208/_00017.html.

Prime Minister's Office of Japan. 2023. "G7 Hiroshima Summit". https://www. kantei.go.jp/g7hiroshima_summit2023/index.html.

Prime Minister's Office of Japan. September 20, 2023. "Prime Minister Fumio Kishida Receives the 2023 Global Goalkeeper Award". https://japan.kantei. go.jp/101_kishida/diplomatic/202309/20award.html.

Qian, Colin and Stephanie Nebehay. October 9, 2020. "China Joins WHO-backed Vaccine Programme COVAX Rejected by Trump". *Reuters*. https:// jp.reuters.com/article/us-health-coronavirus-china-covax/china-joins-who-backed-vaccine-programme-covax-rejected-by-trump-idUSKBN26U027.

Results Japan. March 4, 2020. "Minutes of the 9th Diet Caucus on International Maternal and Child Nutrition Progress toward Tokyo Nutrition

Summit 2020". http://resultsjp.org/wp/wp-content/uploads/2020/03/ Minutes_No9_Diet-Caucus_on_International-Maternal-and-Child-Nutrition_ 20200304.pdf.

Rio Tomonoh Official Site. October 15, 2022. "Daily Activity Report". https:// tomonoh.net/activity-report185/.

Rischbieth, Amanda, George Serafeim, Katie Trinh. 2021. "Accounting for Product Impact in the Pharmaceuticals Industry". *Harvard Business School Working Paper*. 21–139, pp. 1–20. https://www.hbs.edu/impact-weighted-accounts/Documents/Accounting%20for%20Product%20Impact%20in%20the%20Pharmaceuticals%20Industry.pdf?csf=1&web=1&e=8Pells.

Rotary International. 2022. "Rotary and the Fight against Polio". https://www. endpolio.org/rotary-and-the-fight-against-polio.

Rouw, Anna, Jennifer Kates, Josh Michaud, and Adam Wexler. February 18, 2021. "COVAX and the United States". KFF. https://www.kff.org/corona virus-covid-19/issue-brief/covax-and-the-united-states/.

Sakamoto, Haruka, Satoshi Ezoe, Kotono Hara, Yui Sekitani, Keishi Abe, Haruhiko Inada, Takuma Kato, Kenichi Komada, Masami Miyakawa, Eiji Hinoshita, Hiroyuki Yamaya, Naoko Yamamoto, Sarah Krull Abe, and Kenji Shibuya. 2018. "Japan's Contribution to Making Global Health Architecture a Top Political Agenda by Leveraging the G7 Presidency". *Journal of Global Health*. Vol. 8, No. 2. https://www.ncbi.nlm.nih.gov/pmc/articles/ PMC6269922/.

Sakamoto, Haruka, Sarah Krull Abeis, and Satoshi Ezoe. October 30, 2020. "Abe's Legacy: Japan's Contribution to Global Health". *BMJ Global Health*. https://blogs.bmj.com/bmjgh/2020/10/30/abes-legacy-jap ans-contribution-to-global-health/.

Saldinger, Adva. July 24, 2018. "A Look at the Global Financing Facility's Goals, Strategies, and Learnings". https://www.devex.com/news/a-look-at-the-glo bal-financing-facility-s-goals-strategies-and-learnings-93165.

Salisbury, Nicole A., Gilbert Asiimwe, Peter Waiswa, Ashley Latimer. 2019. "Operationalising the Global Financing Facility (GFF) Model: The Devil Is in the Detail". *BMJ Global Health*. Vol. 4, No. 2, pp. 1–3.

Sands, Peter. July 14, 2023. "Japan's Fight Against TB Can Be a Roadmap for Pandemic Preparedness". The Global Fund. https://www.theglobal fund.org/en/opinion/2023/2023-07-14-japans-fight-against-tb-can-be-a-roadmap-for-pandemic-preparedness/.

Sankei Biz. August 27, 2020. "Komeito Leader Yamaguchi Urges Japan's Partic-ipation in COVAX". https://www.sankeibiz.jp/macro/news/200827/mca 2008271424018-n1.htm.

Sanofi Pasteur. 2019. "Imovax Polio". https://e-mr.sanofi.co.jp/-/media/ EMS/Conditions/eMR/leaflet/pdf/IPV_19_08_0169.pdf.

Sato, Tatsuya and Naoki Matsuyama. April 20, 2021. "SDF Helping Army in Philippines in ODA Context". *Asahi Shimbun*. https://www.asahi.com/ajw/articles/14334087.

Save the Children. 2018. "The Global Financing Facility: An Opportunity to Get It Right". https://resourcecentre.savethechildren.net/document/global-financing-facility-opportunity-get-it-right.

Save the Children. April 22, 2022. "9 Million People Die Every Year from Conditions That Should Be Addressed by Their Health System. What Can Be Done to Change This?". https://www.savethechildren.net/blog/9-million-people-die-every-year-conditions-should-be-addressed-their-health-system-what-can-be.

Save the Children Japan. 2021. "Save the Children Japan Annual Report 2020". https://www.savechildren.or.jp/news/publications/download/2020_SCJ_AR_English.pdf.

Save the Children Japan. July 3, 2023. "For the Sake of All Women and Children's Health: What Is the Role of the Global Financing Facility?". https://www.savechildren.or.jp/sp/news/index.php?d=4200.

Science Japan. January 6, 2022. "Solving Global Health Issues: Taking on the Challenge through Collaboration with Partners around the World: Interview with Mihoko Kashiwakura, Head of East Asia Relations, Bill & Melinda Gates Foundation". https://sj.jst.go.jp/stories/2022/s0106-01p.html.

Seidelmann, Lisan, Myria Koutsoumpa, Frederik Federspiel, and Mit Philips. 2020. "The Global Financing Facility at Five: Time for a Change?" *Sexual and Reproductive Health Matters*. Vol. 28, No. 2, pp. 1–8.

Shaw, Rajib and Anjula Gurtoo, eds. 2022. *Global Pandemic and Human Security: Technology and Development Perspective*. Singapore: Springer.

Shibata, Nana. March 28, 2020. "Abe Says Japan Aims to Approve Avigan as Coronavirus Treatment". *Nikkei Asia*. https://asia.nikkei.com/Spotlight/Coronavirus/Abe-says-Japan-aims-to-approve-Avigan-as-coronavirus-treatment.

Shibuya, Kenji, Chorh Chuan Tan, Asaph Young Chun, and Gabriel M. Leung. 2022. "Global Human Security in the Post–COVID-19 Era: The Rising Role of East Asia". *PLOS Medicine*. Vol. 19, No. 7, pp. 1–11.

Shimojo, Hiroto. 1984. "Poliomyelitis Control in Japan". *Reviews of Infectious Diseases*. Vol. 6, Supplement 2, pp. 427–430.

Shinozaki, Natsuki. September 6, 2019. "Japan and China in Africa: From Competition to Collaboration". *NHK News*. https://www3.nhk.or.jp/nhkworld/en/news/backstories/662/.

Shionogi. 2022. "Mother to Mother SHIONOGI Project". https://www.shionogi.com/global/en/sustainability/society/social-contribution-activities/mtom.html.

Shiroyama, Hideaki, ed. 2020. *Global Health Governance*. Tokyo: Toshindo Publishing.

Siddiqi, Sameen, Awad Mataria, Katherine D. Rouleau, and Meesha Iqbal, eds. 2022. *Making Health Systems Work in Low and Middle Income Countries: Textbook for Public Health Practitioners*. Cambridge: Cambridge University Press.

Simpson, Diane M., Nahad Sadr-Azodi, Taufiq Mashal, Wrishmeen Sabawoon, Ajmal Pardis, Arshad Quddus, Carmen Garrigos, Sherine Guirguis, Syed Sohail Zahoor Zaidi, Shahzad Shaukat, Salmaan Sharif, Humayan Asghar, and Stephen C. Hadler. 2014. "Polio Eradication Initiative in Afghanistan, 1997-2013". *Journal of Infectious Diseases*. Vol. 210, No. 1, pp. 162–172.

Slingsby, B. T. and Kiyoshi Kurosawa. 2013. "The Global Health Innovative Technology (GHIT) Fund: Financing Medical Innovations for Neglected Populations". *Lancet Global Health*. Vol. 1, No. 4, pp. 184–185.

SORA Technology. 2022. "About Us". https://www.toyota-tsusho.com/eng lish/press/detail/211217_005879.html.

Soucat, Agnès and Richard Gregory. 2022. "Understanding the Global Health Architecture". In Siddiqi, Sameen, Awad Mataria, Katherine D. Rouleau, and Meesha Iqbal, eds. 2022. *Making Health Systems Work in Low and Middle Income Countries: Textbook for Public Health Practitioners*. Cambridge: Cambridge University Press, pp. 545–562.

Stop TB Partnership. 2022. "Securing the Finances to Save Lives in Africa from Tuberculosis". https://www.stoptb.org/event/ticad-8-official-side-event.

Subramanian, Samanth. August 13, 2020. "Biometric Tracking Can Ensure Billions Have Immunity Against Covid-19". *Bloomberg*. https://www.bloomb erg.com/features/2020-covid-vaccine-tracking-biometric/.

Sugiyama, Haruko, Ayaka Yamaguchi, and Hiromi Murakami. 2013. *Japan's Global Health Policy: Developing a Comprehensive Approach in a Period of Economic Stress*. Edited by Katherine E. Bliss. New York: Rowman & Littlefield Publishers.

Sumitomo Chemical. 2022. "Sumitomo Chemical's Initiatives to Counter Malaria". https://www.sumitomo-chem.co.jp/english/sustainability/social_ contributions/olysetnet/initiative/.

Sun, Lena H. January 18, 2017. "New Global Coalition Launched to Create Vaccines, Prevent Epidemic". *Washington Post*. https://www.washingto npost.com/news/to-your-health/wp/2017/01/18/new-global-coalition-lau nched-to-create-new-vaccines-prevent-epidemics/.

Sunaga, Kazuto. 2004. "The Reshaping of Japan's Official Development Assistance (ODA) Charter". *Discussion Paper on Development Assistance*. No. 3, pp. 1–31.

Suntory. 2022. "The Suntory Group's 7 Sustainability Themes". https://www.suntory.com/csr/themes/health/.

Suzuki, Kazuto. February 26, 2021. "Japan's Vaccine Strategy". *The Diplomat.* https://thediplomat.com/2021/02/japans-vaccine-strategy/.

Swinney, David C. and Michael P. Pollastri, eds. 2019. *Neglected Tropical Diseases: Drug Discovery and Development.* Weinheim: Wiley-VCH.

Sysmex. April 26, 2021. "Dedicated to Eliminating Malaria through the Development of Diagnostic Devices". https://www.sysmex.co.jp/en/stories/210 426_02.html.

Szántó, Diana. 2020. *Politicising Polio: Disability, Civil Society and Civic Agency in Sierra Leone.* Singapore: Palgrave Macmillan.

Szechenyi, Nicholas and Joseph S. Bermudez Jr. April 23, 2020. "Japan's Response to Covid-19: A Work in Progress". *CSIS Commentary.* https://www.csis.org/analysis/japans-response-covid-19-work-progress.

Tadokoro, Ryuko. June 13, 2018. "Former Health Minister Supports Compensation for Forced Sterilization Victims". *Mainichi Shimbun.* https://mainichi.jp/english/articles/20180613/p2a/00m/0na/002000c.

Takahashi, Motoki. 2017. "Changes in TICADs and the World: The Role of Japan in African Development Reconsidered". *Africa Report.* No. 55, pp. 47–61.

Takatsu, T., I. Tagaya, and M. Hirayama. 1973. "Poliomyelitis in Japan during the Period 1962-68 after the Introduction of Mass Vaccination with Sabin Vaccine". *Bulletin of World Health Organization.* Vol. 49, No. 2, pp. 129–137.

Takeda. April 19, 2022. "Takeda Announces Approval of Nuvaxovid® COVID-19 Vaccine for Primary and Booster Immunization in Japan". https://www.takeda.com/newsroom/newsreleases/2022/takeda-announces-approval-of-nuvaxovid-covid-19-vaccine-for-primary-and-booster-immunization-in-japan/.

Takuma, Kayo. 2020. *Jinrui to Yamai (Humankind and Diseases).* Tokyo: Chuokoron-Shinsha.

Takuma, Kayo. September 30, 2020. "Japan Leading Global Health Governance". *East Asia Forum.* https://www.eastasiaforum.org/2020/09/30/japan-leading-global-health-governance/.

Teshirogi, Isao. April 16, 2021. "Significance of Purely Domestically Developed COVID-19 Vaccines in Light of National Security". Federation of Pharmaceutical Manufacturers' Associations of JAPAN (FPMAJ). https://www.kantei.go.jp/jp/singi/kenkouiryou/iyakuhin/dai4/siryou1-2.pdf.

The Access to Medicine Foundation. 2022. *Access to Medicine Index 2022 Methodology.* Amsterdam: The Netherlands.

The Diet Task Force for Eliminating Neglected Tropical Diseases (NTDs). 2021. "Proposal Commitments by the Government of Japan during the 'Global Summit on Malaria and Neglected Tropical Diseases

(Kigali Summit)'". https://jagntd.org/wp-content/uploads/2021/06/Pol icy-recommendations-for-Kigali-Summit-eng.pdf.

The Global Fund. 2022. "The Global Fund to Fight AIDS, Tuberculosis and Malaria". https://www.theglobalfund.org/en/.

The Global Fund. August 27, 2022. "Global Fund Applauds Japan's Major Commitment to Help End AIDS, Tuberculosis and Malaria and Strengthen Systems for Health". https://www.theglobalfund.org/en/news/2022/ 2022-08-27-global-fund-applauds-japans-major-commitment-to-help-end-aids-tuberculosis-and-malaria-and-strengthen-systems-for-health/.

The Global Fund. 2023. "Government and Public Donors: Japan". https:// www.theglobalfund.org/en/government/profiles/japan/.

The Government of Japan. June 16, 2023. "Impact Investing in Global Health: Japan's Commitment as a Frontrunner". *KIZUNA*. https://www.japan.go. jp/kizuna/2023/06/impact_investing_in_global_health.html.

The Guardian. April 13, 2016. "'Like Entering a Prison': Japan's Leprosy Sufferers Reflect on Decades of Pain". https://www.theguardian.com/ world/2016/apr/14/like-entering-a-prison-japans-leprosy-sufferers-sue-gov ernment-for-decades-of-pain.

The Japanese Government. 2023. "Japan's International Cooperation for Global Health". *Highlighting Japan*. https://www.gov-online.go.jp/pdf/hlj/202 30101/hlj202301_24-25_Japans_International_Cooperation_for_Global_ Health.pdf.

The UK Government. 2012. "London Declaration on Neglected Tropical Diseases". https://assets.publishing.service.gov.uk/government/uploads/sys tem/uploads/attachment_data/file/67443/NTD_20Event_20-_20London_ 20Declaration_20on_20NTDs.pdf.

The UK Government. June 22, 2022. "Poliovirus Detected in Sewage from North and East London". https://www.gov.uk/government/news/poliov irus-detected-in-sewage-from-north-and-east-london.

TICAD Monitor.org. 2022. "TICAD 8 Tunis Plan of Actions: Actions for Imple-mentation of TICAD 8 Tunis Plan of Actions". https://ticad-monitor.org/ wp-content/uploads/ENG-TICAD-8-Tunis-Plan-of-Actions.pdf.

Tokyo Shimbun. April 23, 2022. "Kishida Shusho no Ichinichi, April 22 (Prime Minister Kishida's Schedule of April 22)". https://www.tokyo-np.co.jp/art icle/173402.

Toyota Tsusho. December 17, 2021. "Toyota Tsusho Delivers First Refrigerated Vaccine Transport Vehicles to the Ghana Ministry of Health". https://www. toyota-tsusho.com/english/press/detail/211217_005879.html.

Uematsu, Yoshika. May 19, 2020. "Dengue Fever Growing Concern in Japan Due to Deadly Mosquito". *Asahi Shimbun*. https://www.asahi.com/ajw/art icles/13385845.

UNAIDS. 2022. "Humanitarian Crisis: War in Ukraine". https://www.unaids.org/en.

United Nations. 2003. "Human Security Now: Protecting and Empowering People". https://digitallibrary.un.org/record/503749?ln=en.

United Nations Children's Fund (UNICEF). November 3, 2011. "The Japanese Government Contributes 23 Million Yen to Pakistan through UNICEF". https://www.unicef.org/tokyo/news/2011/Nov-3.

United Nations Children's Fund (UNICEF). December 10, 2011. "The Japanese Government Implemented 716 Million Yen Support for Polio Eradication in Afghanistan through the UNICEF". https://www.unicef.org/tokyo/news/2011/Dec-10.

United Nations Children's Fund (UNICEF). December 11, 2012. "The Japanese Government Pledged 13 Million Dollars for Polio Eradication and Diseases Prevention in Afghanistan". https://www.unicef.org/tokyo/news/2012/Dec-11.

United Nations Children's Fund (UNICEF). February 9, 2014. "The Japanese Government Decided on Support of 12 Million Dollars for Polio Eradication and Diseases Prevention Through the UNICEF". https://www.unicef.org/tokyo/news/2014/Feb-9.

United Nations Children's Fund (UNICEF). November 17, 2014. "The Japanese Government Implements 562 Million Yen Support for Polio Eradication in Pakistan". https://www.unicef.org/tokyo/news/2014/Nov-17.

United Nations Children's Fund (UNICEF). February 17, 2016. "The Japanese Government Decided on Support of 1.748 Billion Yen for Diseases Prevention of Children in Afghanistan through the UNICEF". https://www.unicef.org/tokyo/news/2016/Feb-17.

United Nations Children's Fund (UNICEF). March 15, 2016. "The Japanese Government Decided on 360 Million Yen Support for Polio Eradication in Pakistan". https://www.unicef.org/tokyo/news/2016/Mar-15.

United Nations Children's Fund (UNICEF). November 29, 2016. "The Japanese Government Decided on 4.4 Million Yen Contribution to IPV Procurement in Support of Polio Eradication in Pakistan". https://www.unicef.org/tokyo/news/2016/japan-renews-commitment-to-support-polio-eradication-in-pakistan-japanese.

United Nations Children's Fund (UNICEF). December 13, 2016. "Government of Japan Commits US$ 12.4 Million to Provide Life-saving Vaccines in Afghanistan". https://www.unicef.org/tokyo/news/2016/government-of-japan-commits-us-12.4-million-to-provide-life-saving-vaccines-and-prevent-the-spread-of-infectious-diseases-in-afghanistan.

United Nations Children's Fund (UNICEF). February 16, 2017. "Japan Gives $33.3 Million in Emergency Funding to Nigeria and Lake Chad Region".

https://www.unicef.org/tokyo/news/2017/japan-gives-33.3-million-in-emergency-funding-to-protect-children-from-polio-in-nigeria-and-lake-chad-region.

United Nations Children's Fund (UNICEF). October 18, 2017. "The Japanese Government Decided on 520 Million Yen Contribution to Polio Eradication in Pakistan". https://www.unicef.org/tokyo/news/2017/japan-provides-520-million-yen-to-assist-pakistans-efforts-for-polio-eradication-japanese.

United Nations Children's Fund (UNICEF). November 17, 2017. "Japan Donates 17.7 Million USD to Provide Life-Saving Vaccines for Children in Afghanistan". https://www.unicef.org/tokyo/news/2017/japan-donates-17.7-million-usd-to-provide-life-saving-vaccines-for-children-in-afghanistan.

United Nations Children's Fund (UNICEF). November 27, 2017. "Japan Donates 17.7 Million USD to Provide Life-Saving Vaccines for Children in Afghanistan". https://www.unicef.org/tokyo/news/2017/japan-donates-17.7-million-usd-to-provide-life-saving-vaccines-for-children-in-afghanistan.

United Nations Children's Fund (UNICEF). November 19, 2018. "The Japanese Government Decided on 510 Million Yen Contribution to OPV Procurement in Support of Polio Eradication in Pakistan". https://www.unicef.org/tokyo/news/2018/japan-provides-510-million-yen-to-assist-pakistans-efforts-for-polio-eradication-new-us-4.6-million-japanese-grant-to-procure-oral-polio-vaccine-japanese.

United Nations Children's Fund (UNICEF). December 3, 2018. "Japan Donates US$9.1 Million to Support Children and Mother's Health in Afghanistan". https://www.unicef.org/afghanistan/press-releases/japan-donates-us91-million-support-children-and-mothers-health-afghanistan.

United Nations Children's Fund (UNICEF). December 4, 2019. "UNICEF Welcomes Japan's USD 7 Million Contribution to Support Children and Mother's Health in Afghan". https://www.unicef.org/tokyo/news/2019/unicef-welcomes-japan%E2%80%99s-usd-7-million-contribution-to-support-children-and-mother%E2%80%99s-health-in-afghan.

United Nations Children's Fund (UNICEF). December 11, 2019. "Japan Renews Support for Polio Eradication Programme in Pakistan". https://www.unicef.org/tokyo/news/2019/japan-renews-support-for-polio-eradication-programme-in-pakistan.

United Nations Children's Fund (UNICEF). November 10, 2020. "Japan Provides Approximately 9 Million USD to Support Children and Mother's Health in Afghanistan". https://www.unicef.org/tokyo/news/2020/press-releases/japan-provides-approximately-9-million-usd-support-children-and-mothers-health.

United Nations Children's Fund (UNICEF). January 27, 2021. "Japan Renews Commitment to Support Polio Eradication Efforts in Pakistan". https://www.unicef.org/tokyo/news/2021/japan-renews-commitment-to-support-polio-eradication-efforts-in-pakistan.

United Nations Children's Fund (UNICEF). December 13, 2021. "Japan Announces New US$ 4.35 Million Grant to Support Polio Programme in Pakistan". https://www.unicef.org/tokyo/news/2021/japan-announces-new-us-435-million-grant-support-polio-programme-pakistan.

United Nations Children's Fund (UNICEF). 2022. "Polio in Egypt". https://www.unicef.org/egypt/polio-egypt.

United Nations Children's Fund (UNICEF). May 19, 2022. "Japan Contributes US$ 10.4 Million to UNICEF Afghanistan for Administration of Essential Vaccines". https://www.unicef.org/tokyo/news/2022/japan-contributes-us-104-million-unicef-afghanistan-administration-essential.

United Nations Children's Fund (UNICEF). December 8, 2022. "Japan Provides US$ 3.87 Million New Grants for Polio Eradication Efforts in Pakistan". https://www.unicef.org/tokyo/news/2022/japan-provides-us-3.87-million-new-grants-polio-eradication-efforts-pakistan.

United Nations Children's Fund (UNICEF). March 26, 2023. "Government of Japan Contributes over US$21 Million for Vaccines and WASH in Afghanistan's Schools". https://www.unicef.org/tokyo/news/2023/government-japan-contributes-over-us-21-million-life-saving-vaccines-and-water-and-sanitation-in-afghanistans-schools.

United Nations Development Programme (UNDP). 2023. "Human Development Index (HDI)". https://hdr.undp.org/data-center/human-development-index#/indicies/HDI.

United Nations Development Programme (UNDP). 2023. "HDI Dataset". https://hdr.undp.org/data-center/human-development-index#/indicies/HDI.

United Nations Industrial Development Organization (UNIDO). 2022. "YAMAHA Clean Water Supply System Improves People's Lives in Rural Areas". http://www.unido.or.jp/en/technology_db/1674/.

Uniting to Combat NTDs. 2022. "Progress". https://unitingtocombatntds.org/en/neglected-tropical-diseases/progress/.

United to Combat NTDs. 2022. "Reaching a Billion". https://www.infontd.org/resource/reaching-billion-ending-neglected-tropical-diseases-gateway-universal-health-coverage.

United to Combat NTDs. 2022. "The Kigali Declaration". https://unitingtocombatntds.org/en/the-kigali-declaration/.

UN News Center. 2022. "Polio Is No Longer Endemic in Nigeria: UN Health Strategy". https://www.un.org/africarenewal/news/polio-no-longer-endemic-nigeria---un-health-agency.

Vledder, Monique. 2014. "The Health Results Innovation Trust Fund (HRITF): A Model of Learning to Improve Value for Money in Health Programs". *Healthcare Research Seminar Series*. https://wdi.umich.edu/wp-content/uploads/Announcement-Vledder-other-schools-v22.pdf.

Wakabayashi, Mami, Satoshi Ezoe, Makiko Yoneda, Yasushi Katsuma, and Hiroyasu Iso. 2021. "Global Landscape of the COVID-19 Vaccination Policy: Ensuring Equitable Access to Quality-Assured Vaccines". *GHM Open*. Vol. 2, No. 1, pp. 44–50.

Walton, David and Daisuke Akimoto. April 7, 2020. "Japan and Coronavirus: Abe Needs to Make Bold Decisions". *The Interpreter*. https://www.lowyin stitute.org/the-interpreter/japan-and-coronavirus-abe-needs-make-bold-dec isions.

White House. May 20, 2023. "G7 Hiroshima Leaders' Communiqué". https://www.whitehouse.gov/briefing-room/statements-releases/2023/05/20/g7-hiroshima-leaders-communique/.

World Bank. July 13, 2015. "Global Financing Facility Launched with Billions Already Mobilized to End Maternal and Child Mortality by 2030". https://www.worldbank.org/en/news/press-release/2015/07/13/global-financing-facility-launched-with-billions-already-mobilized-to-end-maternal-and-child-mortality-by-2030.

World Bank. December 13, 2017. "World Bank and WHO: Half the World Lacks Access to Essential Health Services, 100 Million Still Pushed into Extreme Poverty Because of Health Expenses". https://www.worldbank.org/en/news/press-release/2017/12/13/world-bank-who-half-world-lacks-access-to-essential-health-services-100-million-still-pushed-into-extreme-poverty-because-of-health-expenses.

World Bank. May 15, 2018. "Japan Trust Fund for Scaling Up Nutrition". https://www.worldbank.org/en/programs/japan-trust-fund-for-scaling-up-nutrition.

World Bank. September 17, 2020. "The World Bank in Japan". https://www.worldbank.org/en/country/japan/overview#1.

World Bank. November 4, 2023. "The Pandemic Fund". https://fiftrustee.worldbank.org/en/about/unit/dfi/fiftrustee/fund-detail/pppr.

World Bank Group. 2019. "Japan Trust Fund for Scaling Up Nutrition (2017–2018 Annual Report)". https://thedocs.worldbank.org/en/doc/985031 597699264502-0090022020/original/JapanTFAnnualReport2019final29 July.pdf.

World Health Organization (WHO). January 4, 2019. "Pakistan and Afghanistan: The Final Wild Poliovirus Bastion". https://www.who.int/news-room/feature-stories/detail/pakistan-and-afghanistan-the-final-wild-poliovirus-bastion.

World Health Organization (WHO). 2021. *World Malaria Report 2021*. https://www.who.int/teams/global-malaria-programme/reports/world-malaria-report-2021.

World Health Organization (WHO). December 10, 2021. "Global Progress against Measles Threatened amidst COVID-19 Pandemic". https://www.who.int/news/item/10-11-2021-global-progress-against-measles-threatened-amidst-covid-19-pandemic.

World Health Organization (WHO). 2022. "COVAX". https://www.who.int/initiatives/act-accelerator/covax.

World Health Organization (WHO). 2022. "Poliomyelitis (Polio)". https://www.who.int/health-topics/poliomyelitis#tab=tab_1.

World Health Organization (WHO). 2022. "Neglected Tropical Diseases". https://www.who.int/health-topics/neglected-tropical-diseases#tab=tab_1.

World Health Organization (WHO). 2022. "Japan: A Champion for Health and Well-Being at All Ages". https://www.who.int/about/funding/contributors/japan.

World Health Organization (WHO). February 17, 2022. "Malawi Declares Polio Outbreak". https://www.afro.who.int/news/malawi-declares-polio-outbreak.

World Health Organization (WHO). May 23, 2022. "Strengthening the Global Architecture for Health Emergency Preparedness, Response and Resilience". https://apps.who.int/gb/ebwha/pdf_files/WHA75/A75_20-en.pdf.

World Health Organization (WHO). October 18, 2022. "Global Leaders Commit US$ 2.6 Billion at World Health Summit to End Polio". https://www.who.int/news/item/18-10-2022-global-leaders-commit-usd-2.6-billion-at-world-health-summit-to-end-polio.

World Health Organization (WHO). May 5, 2023. "Statement on the Fifteenth Meeting of the IHR (2005) Emergency Committee on the COVID-19 Pandemic". https://www.who.int/news/item/05-05-2023-statement-on-the-fifteenth-meeting-of-the-international-health-regulations-(2005)-emergency-committee-regarding-the-coronavirus-disease-(covid-19)-pandemic.

World Health Organization (WHO). September 7, 2023. "Polio: As of Today, the World's Only Public Health Emergency of International Concern". https://www.emro.who.int/polio-eradication/news/polio-as-of-today-the-worlds-only-public-health-emergency-of-international-concern.html.

World Health Organization (WHO). December 19, 2023. "COVID-19 Vaccinations Shift to Regular Immunization as COVAX Draws to a Close". https://www.who.int/news/item/19-12-2023-covid-19-vaccinations-shift-to-regular-immunization-as-covax-draws-to-a-close.

Xu, Xianfen. 2013. "Japan's Official Development Assistance (ODA) Policy Towards China: The Role of Emotional Factors". *Journal of Contemporary East Asia Studies*. Vol. 2, No. 1, pp. 77–94.

Yegorov, Oleg. 21 January 2021. "How the USSR Helped Japan Defeat a Deadly Virus". *Russia Beyond*. https://www.rbth.com/science-and-tech/333327-ussr-japan-polio-vaccine.

Yoneyama, Tetsuo, Takashi Fujiwara, Yoko Yokota, Yoshimi Takemika, and Akio Hagiwara. 1995. "Characterization of a Wild Poliovirus Type 3 Isolated in Japan in 1993". *Japanese Journal of Medical Science and Biology*. Vol. 48, No. 1, pp. 61–70.

Yotsu, Rie R., Yuji Miyamoto, Shuichi Mori, Manabu Ato, Mariko Sugawara-Mikami, Sayaka Yamaguchi, Masashi Yamazaki, Motoaki Ozaki, and Norihisa Ishii. October 21, 2022. "Hansen's Disease (Leprosy) in Japan, 1947–2020: An Epidemiologic Study During the Declining Phase to Elimination". *International Journal of Infectious Diseases*. https://www.ijidonline.com/article/S1201-9712(22)00565-3/fulltext.

# INDEX